MAXIMIZE YOUR MALE HORMONES

SYMPTOMS, CAUSES, AND TREATMENTS OF MEN'S MOST COMMON HEALTH DISORDERS

PAMELA WARTIAN SMITH, MD, MPH, MS

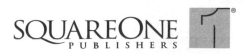

SQUAREONE
PUBLISHERS

EDITOR: Erica Shur
COVER DESIGNER & TYPESETTER: Gary A. Rosenberg

Square One Publishers

115 Herricks Road • Garden City Park, NY 11040

(516) 535-2010 • (877) 900-BOOK

www.squareonepublishers.com

Library of Congress Cataloging-in-Publication Data

Names: Smith, Pamela Wartian, author.
Title: Maximize your male hormones : symptoms, causes, and treatments of
    men's most common health disorders / Pamela Wartian Smith, MD, MPH, MS.
Description: Garden City Park, NY : Square One Publishers, [2023] |
    Includes bibliographical references and index. | Summary: "When there is
    an overproduction or under-production of any of our hormones, we can
    experience a host of serious health disorders. The problem is few of us
    ever connect these issues with our hormones. And while men may be
    familiar with testosterone. Maximize Your Male Hormones, a clear guide
    for men to understand, identify, and treat the many common sources of
    these ailments "— Provided by publisher.
Identifiers: LCCN 2022039376 | ISBN 9780757005152 (paperback) | ISBN
    9780757055157 (ebook)
Subjects: LCSH: Men—Health and hygiene—Popular works. |
    Men—Diseases—Popular works. | Hormone therapy—Popular works.
Classification: LCC RA777.8 .S6556 2023 | DDC 613/.04234—dc23/eng/20220912
LC record available at https://lccn.loc.gov/2022039376

Printed in the United States of America

10   9   8   7   6   5   4   3   2   1

Contents

Part III   Hormone Replacement Therapy

To my husband, Christopher,
who is the love of my life.
Thank you for sharing me with my patients
and the literary world.
Your intelligence, patience, and kindness
bring joy to all around you.

Acknowledgements

To the courageous pioneers of hormone replacement therapy that I have had the privilege to work with as well as educate, who at great personal cost have continued to advance an Anti-Aging Precision Medicine approach to healthcare.

To the compounding pharmacists who have devoted their time, efforts, and personal investment into helping their patients have a customized approach to their healthcare.

To Rudy Shur, the best publisher an author could ever ask for.

To Erica Shur, an editor extraordinaire.

Introduction

How would you like to live to be a healthy 100 years of age? Well, perhaps you can. We now have the scientific means to help you live to be at least 100. However, to live to that age, requires you to be hormonally and nutritionally balanced. Yes, hormones are just as important for men as they are for women. My goal in writing this book is to provide you with hormonal and nutritional tips in order to stay healthy and prevent disease. The objective is also to help you maintain sexual interest and function throughout your lifetime.

All the hormones in the body are a symphony. Much like an orchestra they must play in tune throughout your life in order for you to have optimal health. Hormonal dysfunction can occur at any age—it is not exclusive to older people. In fact, we are now starting to see low testosterone levels in men at younger and younger ages. For example, if you have heart disease, diabetes, weight gain, or erectile dysfunction, it is likely that these diseases are related, in part, to hormonal dysfunction.

Treatments for these kinds of ailments (or any hormonal abnormality, for that matter) may involve hormone replacement therapy (HRT), change in diet, exercise, and/or nutritional therapies. In the past, no matter what your symptoms or hormonal levels were, every man would receive the same one-size-fits-all treatment. Today, medicine has changed, and the science is here to customize and individualize your healthcare.

Medicine is at a crossroads. Now, instead of just treating the symptoms of a disease, a new model of medicine has emerged that looks at the underlying cause of the problem. For example: why might a person suffer from depression? Antidepressants are wonderful medications—if you need them. Their purpose is to treat the symptoms of depression—not to uncover the cause of depression. In the new specialty of Precision Medicine/Anti-Aging Medicine, the reason why a person has depression would be examined. Depression may be a symptom of hypothyroidism, which is low thyroid function. Perhaps, it may be the result of the sufferer's body no longer making enough testosterone. A number of studies have reported a link between low testosterone and depression. In older men with low testosterone, raising testosterone levels can have an antidepressant effect. There may be a neurotransmitter imbalance or perhaps the GI tract is not functioning optimally. There are many different factors that can cause depression, and Precision/Anti-Aging Medicine aims to find and alleviate the cause instead of only treating the various symptoms. Just because two people are suffering the same problems does not mean they should receive the same treatment. This specialty recognizes this concept and treats patients accordingly. To find a Precision/Anti-Aging specialist, see the Resources section of this book.

The pages of this text will explore the intricate web of your body's hormonal system which is relevant to men of all ages, whether you are 27, 47, or 77 years of age.

Part I of the book explores the different hormones in your body, their functions, and the various side effects that can occur if these hormones are not at optimal levels. Additionally, the importance of hormonal levels and the ratio between them will be revealed. You will also learn the different causes that can create hormonal imbalances, which may help you eliminate an issue before it becomes a problem. The perfect levels of all your hormones are needed for you to achieve optimal health. For example, too much testosterone is just as problematic as too little of this important hormone in your body.

Part I, The Hormones. I have organized this section in the order I felt would be most useful to you, the reader. While the order of importance for every man may be different, understanding each hormone is key.

Part II, Ailments and Problems, focuses on the most common ailments and problems that arise from hormonal imbalances, such as erectile dysfunction (ED), male infertility, diabetes, benign prostatic hypertrophy (BPH), and prostate cancer, to name a few. You'll learn that even diseases that seemingly have nothing to do with hormones—like heart disease and osteoporosis (yes men can lose bone structure at about the same rate as women once they lose hormonal function) —can be affected by a hormonal imbalance. Low testosterone does not just lead to loss of muscle strength and mass. Bones are affected as well. Consequently, keeping your hormones at optimal levels is beneficial in preventing a wide array of health disorders, even ones you wouldn't suspect.

Part III focuses on hormone replacement therapy. Twelve reasons you should consider compounded hormone replacement therapy will be discussed. In addition, this section of the book examines, at length, the four big reasons you should consider HRT: 1. Hormones help to maintain cognitive function. In one study, men with low testosterone were on average 48 percent more likely to develop Alzheimer's disease than those with normal levels. 2. Hormones aid in preventing and are adjunct therapies for heart disease. Lower levels of testosterone are associated with higher rates of cardiovascular disease. 3. Hormones are of benefit in keeping your blood sugar and weight optimal. Men with lower testosterone are more likely to have insulin resistance, diabetes, and abdominal obesity. 4. Hormones are important for sexual function and interest. Low testosterone contributes to erectile dysfunction and affects the brain which leads to loss of libido. Moreover, part III explores how to get started should you decide HRT is the option for you. Different ways to have your hormone levels measured are likewise discussed. Finally, you will learn how proper nutrition can benefit your health and boost the effects of hormone replacement therapy.

Fortunately, you do not have to suffer in silence like your fathers did! Science can help us. Not only can you have your symptoms improve or even resolve, but you now have a better chance of helping maintain your vision, memory, mobility, and sexual function. This is not "Star Trek" medicine. It is here and available now. You too can have individualized and customized care. This book will help you discover how.

PART I

Hormones

INTRODUCTION

The hormones in your body are a key component of your overall health. A hormone is a chemical substance produced in the body that controls and regulates the activity of certain cells or organs. All of the hormones in your body interact with each other. They are a web, a symphony that must play in tune in order for you to feel great and be healthy.

This part of the book examines many of the hormones in the body. Your sex hormones, testosterone, progesterone, estrogen (yes men make estrogen), and DHEA will be explored. Your sex hormones interact with cortisol (your stress hormone) and other hormones in the body. These hormones are all made by pregnenolone, your hormone of memory. Hormones literally play as a symphony in your body. If your hormonal symphony is playing in tune, you feel fabulous and have sexual interest and function. If your hormones are not balanced (playing out of tune), you will experience symptoms and increase your risk of developing various diseases, such as obesity, diabetes, heart disease, and high blood pressure.

Additionally, these hormones all interact with your thyroid hormone which regulates many of the functions in your body. Just like the ratio between your sex hormones is important, thyroid levels that are too high or too low can have serious consequences, which will also be explored in Part I of this book.

Your hormone levels change throughout your lifetime. The amount of hormones your body makes and the degree of fluctuation or change in hormone levels are important. There are many things that influence how much of a hormone is made. For example, if you are stressed, take an antibiotic, or are near toxins, have an unhealthy diet, exercise too much or not enough, or take too few or too many vitamins, the amount of hormones that your body produces will be affected. The aging process also affects hormone production.

Let us begin our hormonal journey.

TESTOSTERONE

Testosterone in males is secreted by the testes. In the adult male, 95 percent of the testosterone that is circulating in the blood is made in the Leydig cells of the testes; 6 to 7 mg a day of testosterone is made in the healthy adult man. The remaining 5 percent of the circulating testosterone is made in the adrenal glands. Testosterone plays many important roles; it is needed for growth, increase in muscle mass, development of the penis, and facial and body hair along with deepening of the male voice. In adults, testosterone has many functions in the body. The making of testosterone is regulated by biofeedback mechanism which can be influenced by physiological, pharmacological, and lifestyle factors. You will also hear the term androgen. Androgens are steroids and include testosterone and androsterone, and DHEA, all of which regulate the growth, development, and function of the male reproductive system.

The liver breaks down testosterone into inactive metabolites that are then excreted via the urine and the skin and into active metabolites: dihydrotestosterone (DHT) and two estrogens (estrone and estradiol). The conversion of testosterone to DHT occurs under the action of three types of 5 alpha-reductase. Testosterone is unable to be stored in the testes.

Consequently, testosterone is found: 2 percent in the bioavailable form in the plasma bound to albumin and sex hormone binding globulin (SHBG), 54 percent is weakly bound to albumin, and 44 percent is bound to sex hormone binding globulin. SHBG may increase with age. Consequently, as hormone levels decline even lower levels may be available for the body to use since more of the hormones may be bound to SHBG. Therefore, it is important to have your healthcare provider also measure SHBG levels in the body. The combination of free and albumin-bound testosterone is what determines the bioavailable amount of testosterone. High levels of estrogen increase the body's production of SHBG in a male. Therefore, high levels of estrogen cause more testosterone to be bound in a male. Signs of feminization may occur.

■ Functions of Testosterone in Your Body

- Builds and maintains muscle mass and strength
- Causes vasorelaxation which lowers vascular pressure
- Helps maintain a powerful immune system
- Improves mood
- Improves oxygen uptake throughout the body
- Increases lean body mass
- Lowers cholesterol
- Maintains libido
- Prevents memory loss
- Reduces body fat mass
- Regulates blood sugar
- Regulates nutrient and energy balance to maintain protein synthesis
- Regulates red blood cell production
- Sperm production

■ Signs and Symptoms of Low Testosterone

- ❏ Anxiety
- ❏ Cognitive decline
- ❏ Decreased ability to concentrate
- ❏ Decreased muscle mass
- ❏ Depression
- ❏ Difficulty achieving and maintaining an erection
- ❏ Hair loss
- ❏ Hot flashes
- ❏ Increase in breast tissue
- ❏ Increase in perceived stress
- ❏ Increased risk of bone loss and bone fracture
- ❏ Infertility
- ❏ Insomnia
- ❏ Irritability

❑ Low blood count (anemia)   ❑ Reduced sperm count

❑ Low sex drive   ❑ Small testicles

❑ Reduced body and facial hair   ❑ Weight gain

❑ Reduced energy

◼ Causes of Low Testosterone

● Aging process

● Alcohol use

  • Physical stress immediately before alcohol use prolongs the reduction in testosterone

  • Alcohol abuse may lead to thyroid and adrenal dysfunction which may further lower testosterone

  • Alcohol abuse can cause high estrogen levels in males

● Cholesterol levels that are too low (most scientist suggest that total cholesterol must be at least 140 mg/dL to make pregnenolone and to make testosterone and the other sex hormones)

● Chronic illness

● Chronic kidney failure

● Diabetes

● Disease of the hypothalamus which produces low gonadotropin-releasing hormone (GnRH)

● Disorders of the pituitary gland

● Elevated prolactin levels due to stress, pituitary tumors (prolactinomas), and medications that can raise prolactin levels

● Genetic disorders such as Klinefelter syndrome, Prader-Willi syndrome, Myotonic dystrophy, Kallman syndrome, and hemochromatosis (hereditary disease that causes your body to absorb too much iron from the food you eat)

● HIV/AIDS

● Hypothyroidism (low thyroid function)

- Infection of the testes
  - Arbodengue
  - Chlamydia
  - COVID-19 (currently being studied)
  - Coxsackie
  - Epstein-Barr
  - Gonorrhea
  - Herpes
  - Marburg virus
  - Mumps

- Injury to the testicles due to trauma or surgery

- Kidney or liver disease

- Lack of exercise

- Medications such as opiates (heroin, morphine, methadone), some anti-depressants, medications for anxiety, some seizure medications, and some antipsychotic drugs, and drugs that may directly affect the testes, such as:
  - Aminoglutethamide
  - Anticonvulsants
  - Barbiturates
  - Cannabinoids
  - Chemotherapy
  - Cimetidine
  - Cyproterone acetate
  - Digoxin
  - Heroin
  - HMG-CoA reductase inhibitors
  - Ketoconazole
  - Methadone
  - Psychotropic drugs
  - Spirnolactone

- Obesity

- Other medications such as aromatase inhibitors

- Temperature
  - Varicocele and hydrocele impair the temperature regulation of the scrotum which keeps the testes at the right temperature
  - Scrotal cooling may be improved by wearing boxer shorts, avoiding tight jeans and long periods of driving

- Vegetarian diets, particularly if low in protein, can increase sex hormone binding globulin (SHBG) which lowers free testosterone, the testosterone available for the body to use.

■ Side Effects of High Testosterone Levels

- Acne
- Aggressive behavior
- Delusions
- Elevated cholesterol
- Euphoria
- Fluid retention with swelling of the legs and feet
- Headaches
- Heart muscle damage
- High blood pressure
- Impaired judgment
- Impotence
- Increase heart hypertrophy (heart enlargement)

- Increased appetite
- Increased risk of blood clots
- Increased risk of heart attack
- Increased risk of stroke
- Insomnia
- Irritability
- Liver disease
- Low sperm counts
- Mood swings
- Prostate enlargement with difficulty urinating
- Shrinking of the testicles
- Weight gain

■ Symptoms of High Testosterone

- ❏ Chest pain or discomfort
- ❏ Cough or urge to cough
- ❏ Difficulty with breathing/ swallowing
- ❏ Fast, pounding, or irregular heartbeat or pulse
- ❏ Groin pain/bladder pain
- ❏ Muscle aches

- ❏ Pain or burning with urination/ frequent urge to urinate
- ❏ Pain or discomfort in the arms, jaw, back, or neck
- ❏ Puffiness or swelling around the eyes, face, lips, or tongue
- ❏ Skin rash, hives, itching
- ❏ Sweating
- ❏ Unusual tiredness or weakness

Testosterone Replacement

Men lose hormones as they age. This process is called andropause. The definition of andropause is an absolute or relative insufficiency of testosterone or its metabolites in relation to the needs of that individual at that time in his life. Depending on the study that you read, between 30 percent to 80 percent of men in their 70s are hypogonadal, meaning that they have low testosterone levels. In fact, half of healthy men between the ages of 50 to 70 years will have a testosterone level below the lowest level seen in healthy men who are 20 to 40 years of age. The following graph depicts the decline of testosterone that occurs with age.

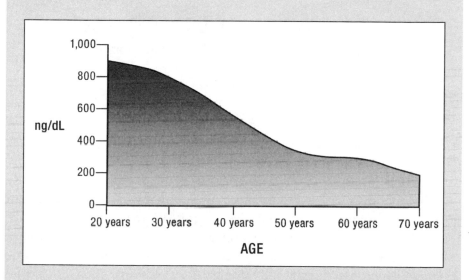

The Massachusetts Male Aging Study showed a 30-year fall in total testosterone in men averaging 48 percent and a decline in free testosterone of 85 percent. There are also seasonal variations in levels of testosterone with peak levels found in the summer and early fall and lower levels in the winter and early spring. A male makes between 4 to 8 mg of testosterone a day and his hormone levels change 4 to 6 times a day.

■ Signs and Symptoms of Andropause

- ❑ Anxiety or nervousness
- ❑ Backache, joint pains, or stiffness
- ❑ Bone loss
- ❑ Decline in physical abilities
- ❑ Decrease in job performance
- ❑ Decreased intensity of orgasms
- ❑ Depression, low or negative mood
- ❑ Elevated cholesterol
- ❑ Fatigue, tiredness, or loss of energy
- ❑ Feeling over-stressed
- ❑ Increased risk of heart disease
- ❑ Increased risk of insulin resistance, diabetes, and metabolic syndrome
- ❑ Irritability, anger, or bad temper
- ❑ Loss of erections or problems during sex
- ❑ Loss of fitness
- ❑ Loss of memory or concentration
- ❑ Loss of sex drive or libido
- ❑ Weight gain

There are many studies in the medical literature revealing that low testosterone levels increase a male's risk of heart disease. One study revealed that men with coronary heart disease that were under the age of 45 had total and free testosterone levels significantly lower than controls. Other studies have shown that blood free testosterone levels were found to be inversely related to carotid intima-media thickness (IMT) and plaque score, which are risk factors for coronary heart disease. Yet another trial revealed that low testosterone levels were found to be associated with atherosclerosis in men. In addition, a recent study revealed that reduced testosterone levels in men with congestive heart failure suggests a poor prognosis and is associated with increased mortality. The same study also revealed that low testosterone levels in men may increase their risk of developing not only coronary heart disease but also metabolic syndrome and type 2 diabetes. Likewise, in males with heart failure, low serum levels of testosterone were associated with an adverse outcome. Furthermore, studies have shown that low testosterone predicts an increase in mortality from cardiovascular disease and an increased risk of death from all causes. In fact, another study revealed that low testosterone levels were associated with an increased risk of all-cause mortality independent of numerous risk factors.

Many trials have shown that low testosterone levels are associated with an increase in insulin resistance, diabetes, and metabolic syndrome, which is a cluster of diseases that increase your risk of heart disease. In fact, since testosterone has been shown to lower blood sugar levels, the Endocrine Society now recommends measurement of testosterone in all male patients with type 2 diabetes. A trial also showed that low total testosterone concentrations are predictive of hypertension (high blood pressure), suggesting total testosterone as a potential biomarker for increased cardiovascular risk.

Testosterone also has a strong effect on memory and concentration. Animal studies suggest that memory loss that occurs with aging is related to testosterone loss and that even the increased expression of amyloid-B-related peptides that occurs with Alzheimer's disease is related to low testosterone levels in men. In one study, the age-related decline in free testosterone predicted age-related decline in visual and verbal memory. Furthermore, another trial revealed that low levels of bioavailable testosterone are a positive predictor of memory loss in men as they age. In a medical trial done in Hong Kong, in men with low bioavailable testosterone levels there was a strong correlation with memory loss/Alzheimer's disease. Likewise, another medical trial, a prospective longitudinal study, revealed that the risk of Alzheimer's disease was decreased by 26 percent for each 10-unit (nmoL/nmoL) increase in free testosterone at 2, 5, and 10 years before the diagnosis of Alzheimer's disease was made. In fact, low testosterone levels have also been associated with mild memory loss that is not related to Alzheimer's disease. Moreover, studies have also shown a correlation between testosterone levels and cognitive abilities, such as spatial performance and mathematical reasoning.

Consequently, testosterone replacement is suggested for males, as they age, if they are candidates for testosterone replacement. See the section on Hormone Replacement Therapy for Males in Part III of this book for a further discussion.

ESTROGEN

The presence of estrogen in males has been known for over 90 years. Males make estrogen from pregnenolone and DHEA. Men make three types of estrogen: estrone (E1), estradiol (E2), and estriol (E3). It is important to measure both estrone and estradiol. Estriol is still experimental. Estradiol has a protective effect on the brain structures in older males. Serum estradiol and testosterone levels have been shown to be lower in men with Alzheimer's disease compared with age-matched controls. Males also need a small amount of estrogen to help maintain bone structure. Androgens, including testosterone, aromatize into estrogens via the enzyme aromatase which is expressed in Leydig cells, seminiferous epithelium, and other male organs. Aromatization is a natural process that the body goes through to maintain homeostasis. Therefore, in men about 15 percent of circulating estrogens derive directly from testicular production with the remainder generated from androgens through peripheral activity of the enzyme aromatase.

Early studies showed E2 binding in numerous male tissues and their main nuclear receptors (ESR1 and ESR2) each show unique distributions and actions in males. Efferent ductules (a network of small ducts that conduct sperm from the testes to the epididymis) and epididymal (where sperm cells mature and are stored) functions are dependent on estrogen signaling through ESR1. Loss of ESR1 or aromatase also produces effects on nonreproductive targets, such as brain, adipose (fat cells), skeletal muscle, bone, cardiovascular, and immune tissues. Evidence also suggests that membrane ESR1 has critical roles in male reproduction. In addition, estrogen signaling has a key role in prostate cancer development and progression. Moreover, estrogen metabolism has been shown to modulate bone density in males.

Recent data from clinical intervention studies indicate that estradiol may be a stronger determinant of adiposity (obesity) than testosterone in men, and even short-term estradiol deprivation contributes to an increase in fat.

■ Functions of Estrogen in Males

- Bone maturation/regulation of bone resorption

- Contributes to spermatogenesis

- Helps maintain memory

- Lipid metabolism

- Promotes the production of sperm

- Regulates gonadotropin feedback

- Regulation of erectile response

■ Signs and Symptoms of Deficiency

❏ Osteopenia/osteoporosis

❏ Cognitive decline

❏ Dyslipidemia (abnormal cholesterol and triglyceride levels)

■ Causes of Estrogen Deficiency

- Addison's disease
    - Exposure to radiation
    - Genetic disorders like Turner syndrome or Klinefelter syndrome
- Infections that affect the sexual organs
    - Histocytosis
    - Human immunodeficiency virus (HIV)
    - Mumps
    - Tuberculosis (TB)
- Iron overload in your blood (hemochromatosis)
- Kidney or liver disease
- Medications may decrease estrogen levels in men and cause estrogen levels to be too low
    - Carbamazepine
    - Chlordiazepoxide
    - Phenobarbital
    - Sucralfate
    - Trazodone
- Overdose of medications that lower estrogen
    - Anastrozole and other aromatase inhibitors
    - Too high a dose of Chrysin (usually used transdermally)
- Nutritional deficiencies
- Obesity
- Pituitary tumor
- Rapid weight loss
- Surgery on the penis or testicles
- Testicles that do not descend

■ Recommended Daily Dosage

Estradiol placement is not suggested in males. Estriol replacement in males is currently only being used in individuals to treat autoimmune encephalitis and multiple sclerosis.

■ Foods That Increase Estrogen Levels

If you would like to boost your estrogen levels naturally, dietary choices may be the answer. Similarly, if your estrogen levels are consistently high, the cause of this issue may be found on your plate. You may be consuming large amounts of foods that are known to increase this hormone in the body, such as the following examples.

Vegetables

Artichoke	Chives	Pea seedlings
Asparagus	Corn	Potato (all kinds)
Bamboo shoots	Cucumber	Pumpkin
Beet	Eggplant	Radish
Bell pepper (red, green,	Garlic	Seaweed
yellow, orange)	Green beans	Shallot
Brussels sprouts	Lettuce	Spinach
Cabbage	Mustard greens	Tomato
Carrot	Okra	Turnip
Cauliflower	Onion	Yam
Celery	Parsley	

Fruits

Apple	Grapefruit	Pear
Apricot	Lemon	Pineapple
Banana	Muskmelon	Plum
Cherry	Orange	Strawberry
Date	Peach	Watermelon
Grape		

Cereals and Grains

Barley	Rice	Wheat (bran, flour,
Corn	Rye	whole)

Legumes (Beans)

Chickpeas	Pea	Soybean
Kidney	Peanut	

Seeds and Nuts

Almond	Pecan	Sesame seed
Cashew	Pine nut	Sunflower seed
Coconut	Pistachio	Walnut

Oils

Coconut	Peanut	Soybean
Corn	Rice bran	Sunflower
Linseed (flaxseed)	Safflower	Walnut
Olive	Sesame seed	Wheat germ

■ Side Effects and Contraindications

Estrogen should not be used in men with prostate or breast cancer even if they have multiple sclerosis or autoimmune encephalitis.

■ Signs and Symptoms of Elevated Levels of Estrogen

- ❏ Bloated or retaining water
- ❏ BPH (benign prostatic hyperplasia)
- ❏ Decreased sex drive/erectile dysfunction
- ❏ Doubled risk of having a CVA (stroke)
- ❏ Erectile dysfunction
- ❏ Fatigue
- ❏ Gynecomastia (enlarged breasts in men)
- ❏ Higher rate of insulin resistance
- ❏ Higher rates of myocardial infarction, peripheral artery disease, and carotid artery stenosis (blockage)
- ❏ Increased rate of rheumatoid arthritis
- ❏ Increased risk of developing prostate cancer
- ❏ Increased risk of heart disease

■ Causes of Elevated Levels of Estrogen

- Antacids: omeprazole, cimetidine

- Antibiotics: sulfas, tetracyclines, penicillins, cefoazolins, erythromycins, quinolones

- Antidepressants: fluoxetine, fluvoxamine, paroxetine, sertraline

- Anti-fungals: miconazole, itraconazole, fluconazole, ketoconazole

- Anti-hypertensive drugs: propranolol, quinidine, amiodarone (also decreases testosterone production), coumadin, methyldopa

- Anti-psychotic medications: Thorazine, haloperidol

- Cholesterol-lowering statins

- Estrogen levels may elevate as men age due to the following:
  - Abuse of alcohol
  - Alteration in liver function
  - Environmental estrogens
  - Foods that may increase estrogen levels (see list on page 16)
  - Grapefruit
  - High dose vitamin E
  - High doses of testosterone
  - Increased aromatase activity

- Medications
  - Pain control medications: NSAIDs, acetaminophen, propoxyphene
  - Recreational drugs: amphetamines, marijuana, cocaine

- Obesity

- Zinc deficiency

■ Ways to Lower High Estrogen Levels In Males

- Anastrozole and other aromatase inhibitors

- Chrysin (usually used transdermally)

- Decrease alcohol intake

- Decrease dose of testosterone
- Decrease intake of estrogen containing foods
- Eating foods that decrease estrogen
- Eating organic foods and avoid environmental estrogens
- Grape seed extract
- High dose vitamin C (also increases testosterone production)

- Lose weight
- Maca
- Niacin
- Resveratrol
- Vitamin K
- Wild nettle root
- Zinc

■ Therapeutic Benefits of Estrogen

Estrogen is important in males for bone structure, cognitive function, and dyslipidemia (abnormal cholesterol and triglycerides level) regulation. As you have seen, it is paramount that a male's estrogen level be optimal, not too low, or too high. This statement is just as true for men as it is for women.

PROGESTERONE

Progesterone is a hormone that is produced in males, and it has many great functions in the body.

■ Functions of Progesterone in Your Body

- Affects adipose tissue
- Affects behavior
- Affects respiratory system
- Blocking of gonadotropin secretion (group of hormones secreted by the pituitary which stimulate the activity of the gonads)

- Calming effect
- Cardioprotective (heart protective)
- Affects the potentiation of GABA
- Helps with myelination

- Immunoprotective (positive affect on the immune system)

- Influences spermiogenesis

- Involved in kidney function

- Neuroprotective

- Progesterone functions as a 5-alpha reductase inhibitor. 5-alpha-reductase inhibitors are a group of drugs that are used in the treatment of an enlarged prostate gland and male pattern hair loss.

- Sleep improvement

There is one common sign/symptom of progesterone deficiency in a male and that is prostate enlargement. There are also no known causes of progesterone deficiency and there is no age-dependent change in serum progesterone concentrations.

Progesterone Replacement

Progesterone replacement is commonly prescribed on the skin. It has also been used as an IV for traumatic brain injury (TBI) and post-CVA (stroke). There are no known side effects or contraindications at this time to progesterone replacement although it is not suggested in people with prostate cancer. If you are prescribed too much progesterone, you may have sexual dysfunction.

■ Therapeutic Benefits of Progesterone

- BPH (benign prostatic hyperplasia)

- Cognitive decline

- Elevated DHT (dihydrotestosterone)

- Multiple sclerosis (MS)

- Post-stroke

- Traumatic brain injury (TBI)
    - Modulates apoptosis, inflammation, oxidative stress, excitotoxicity
    - Protects and rebuilds blood-brain barrier
    - Decreases development of cerebral edema (swelling of the brain)

- Limits cellular necrosis (cell death)
- Used in conjunction with vitamin D

DHEA

DHEA is made by the adrenal glands with a small amount being created by the brain and skin. DHEA makes estrogen and testosterone. DHEA production declines with age, starting in the late twenties. In men, plasma DHEAS concentrations decrease by an average of 1 percent to 4 percent per year between the ages of 40 and 80 years. By the age of 70, the body only makes about one-fourth of the amount that it made earlier. Furthermore, DHEA levels change if the patient is stressed long-term. When the patient is first stressed, DHEA levels increase. Overtime, if the patient remains stressed, DHEA levels become low.

Functions of DHEA in Your Body

- Anti-inflammatory
- Antioxidant
- Decreases age-related skin atrophy, stimulating procollagen, and sebum production
- Decreases allergic reactions by attenuating T helper 2 allergic inflammation
- Decreases formation of fatty deposits
- Helps the body repair itself and maintain tissues
- Helps you deal with stress
- Increases bone growth
- Increases cognition
- Increases growth hormone levels
- Increases lean body mass
- Increases nitric oxide
- Increases sense of well-being

- Lowers cholesterol

- Lowers triglycerides

- Prevents advanced glycation end-products (AGE) formation

- Prevents blood clots

- Promotes weight loss by reducing body fat

- Protective in asthma by reducing airway hyperactivity and eosinophilia which is a condition in which the eosinophil count in the peripheral blood is high. This occurs in allergic conditions and in asthma.

- Reduces blood sugar, reduces spikes in blood sugar, and decreases rate of insulin resistance

- Supports the immune system (In the elderly, DHEA exerts an immunomodulatory action, increasing the number of monocytes, T cells expressing T-cell receptor gamma/delta (TCRγδ) and natural killer (NK) cells.)

■ Signs and Symptoms of DHEA Deficiency

- ❑ Decreased energy
- ❑ Decreased muscle strength
- ❑ Difficulty dealing with stress
- ❑ Increased risk of infection
- ❑ Irritability
- ❑ Joint soreness
- ❑ Weight gain

■ Causes of DHEA Deficiency

- Aging process
- Andropause
- Prolonged stress
- Smoking (nicotine inhibits the production of 11-beta-hydroxylase, an enzyme needed to make DHEA)

■ Recommended Daily Dosage

- According to test results, most common dosage is 10 to 100 mg orally.

- May be used orally or transdermally (applied to the skin) but is mostly commonly used orally. It is best if used SR (E4M) but the GI tract needs to be healthy for optimal release.

■ Other Sources of DHEA

The level of DHEA commonly normalizes in a younger patient as cortisol normalizes. Therefore, in younger patients DHEA is not always replaced. It is important to always fix the cause of the problem, which is usually long-term stress.

■ Side Effects and Contraindications

DHEA replacement therapy is contraindicated in patients with a history of hormonally related cancers such as prostate or male breast cancer.

■ Signs and Symptoms of Elevated Levels of DHEA

❏ Acne	❏ Facial hair	❏ Mood changes
❏ Anger	❏ Fatigue	❏ Restless sleep
❏ Deeper voice	❏ Insomnia	❏ Sugar cravings
❏ Depression	❏ Irritability	❏ Weight gain

■ Therapeutic Benefits of DHEA

- Allergy
- Andropause
- Asthma
- Cognition
- Coronary heart disease
- Depression
- Hypercholesterolemia (high cholesterol)
- Hypertriglyceridemia (high triglycerides)
- Insomnia
- Insulin resistance/diabetes
- Lupus
- Osteopenia/osteoporosis (bone loss)
- Post-traumatic stress disorder (PTSD)
- Rheumatoid arthritis
- Sexual dysfunction
- Stress
- Weight loss
- Ankylosing spondylitis

■ Causes of Elevated Levels of DHEA

- Adrenal tumor
- Long-term stress

- Patient is prescribed a dose of DHEA that is too high

CORTISOL

Cortisol is one of the only hormones in your body that increases with age. It is also one of your sex hormones. Like DHEA, cortisol is made by your adrenal glands, which make all your sex hormones after andropause. Cortisol levels are regulated by the adrenocorticotropic hormone (ACTH), which is synthesized by the pituitary in response to the corticotropin-releasing hormone (CRH). CRH is released by the hypothalamus. Cortisol is commonly known as the "stress hormone" due to its involvement in your response to stress.

Low levels of cortisol are characterized as hypocortisolism, hypoadrenalism, or adrenal fatigue. High levels of cortisol are characterized as hypercortisolism or hyperadrenalism. When no cortisol is produced, Addison's disease is indicated. When extremely high levels of cortisol are produced, Cushing's disease is indicated.

■ Functions of Cortisol in Your Body

- Acts as an anti-inflammatory
- Affects pituitary/thyroid/ adrenal system
- Balances blood sugar
- Balances DHEA
- Controls weight
- Improves mood and thoughts
- Influences estrogen/ testosterone ratio

- Participates with aldosterone in sodium reabsorption
- Promotes good sleep hygiene
- Regulates bone turnover rate
- Regulates immune system response
- Supports protein synthesis
- Regulates the stress reaction

Abnormal cortisol levels that are too high or too low can be associated with many medical conditions.

■ Conditions Associated With Abnormal Levels of Cortisol

- Alzheimer's disease
- Anorexia nervosa
- Chronic fatigue syndrome
- Coronary heart disease
- Depression
- Diabetes
- Exacerbations of multiple sclerosis
- Fibromyalgia
- Generalized memory loss
- Heart disease
- Impotence

- Infertility
- Insulin resistance
- Irritable bowel syndrome (IBS)
- Osteoporosis
- Panic disorders
- Post-traumatic stress disorder (PTSD)
- Prostate cancer
- Rheumatoid arthritis
- Sleep disorders
- Weight gain

There is a strong interrelationship between activation of the hypothalamic-pituitary-adrenal (HPA) axis and energy balance. Individuals with abdominal obesity tend to have elevated cortisol levels. Furthermore, stress and glucocorticoids (steroid hormones) act to control both food intake and energy expenditure. Glucocorticoids are known to increase the consumption of foods high in fat and sugar in animals and humans. High cortisol individuals eat more in response to stress than low cortisol, leading to increased food intake and reduced energy expenditure; thus, a predisposition to obesity. Therefore, cortisol responsiveness may be used as a marker to identify people who are at risk of weight gain and subsequent obesity.

The optimal method of measuring cortisol for the purposes of balancing your hormones (not for the diagnosis of Addison's disease or Cushing's disease) is salivary testing. An assay for cortisol levels will not be as accurate if you have been on steroids within the last thirty days. Contact your healthcare provider to discuss steroid use and cortisol measurement if you are taking prescription steroids. If you require long-term steroid treatment for another medical problem, your doctor can take this information into account when interpreting the results of the saliva test. If you are on steroids short-term, then usually your healthcare provider will not have you do saliva testing within one month of your using a prescription for a steroid medication (such as an asthma inhaler).

When you are stressed, your cortisol levels increase. When you are stressed for a long time, then your cortisol levels can actually become too low. You require cortisol, however, to survive. Therefore, when cortisol becomes too low, your body will take pregnenolone to make cortisol, no matter what age you are, even if it means depleting your body of pregnenolone.

When your adrenal glands do not produce enough cortisol, your body is in a state of emergency, and consequently you do not feel well. You may turn to coffee, soft drinks, or sugar as a source of energy, but this will only make the situation worse. Consuming any of these items will temporarily make you feel better or more energetic, but the negative effects far outweigh the temporary fix. If your adrenal glands stay stimulated when they are in a state of emergency, they may weaken and "burn out." When this happens, your cortisol and DHEA levels will drop. This is called adrenal fatigue, or hypoadrenalism.

If the adrenals become totally depleted, this condition is called Addison's disease. If you have Addison's disease, your body makes no cortisol at all. Adrenal fatigue is not a total depletion of cortisol, but it does bring cortisol levels down low enough to prevent optimal functioning of the body. Adrenal fatigue is one of the most pervasive and underdiagnosed syndromes of modern society. A deficiency of cortisol that is not Addison's disease is usually caused by stress.

■ Signs and Symptoms of Adrenal Fatigue (Cortisol Deficiency)

❏ Allergies (environmental sensitivities and chemical intolerance)

❏ Decreased immunity

❏ Decreased sexual interest

❏ Digestive problems

❏ Drug addiction

❏ Emotional imbalances

❏ Emotional paralysis

❏ Fatigue

❏ Feeling overwhelmed

❏ General feeling of "unwellness"

- ❑ Hypoglycemia (low blood sugar)
- ❑ Increased risk of alcoholism and drug addiction
- ❑ Lack of stamina
- ❑ Loss of motivation or initiative
- ❑ Low blood pressure
- ❑ Poor healing of wounds
- ❑ Progressively poorer athletic performance
- ❑ Sensitivity to light
- ❑ Unresponsive hypothyroidism (low thyroid function that doesn't respond to treatment)

■ Causes of Low Cortisol

- ● Chronic inflammation
- ● Chronic pain
- ● Depression
- ● Dysbiosis
- ● Hypoglycemia
- ● Long-term stress
- ● Nutritional deficiencies
- ● Overly aggressive exercise without nutritional support
- ● Poor sleep
- ● Severe allergies
- ● Toxic exposure

If your cortisol level is too low due to adrenal fatigue from long-term stress, begin your therapy with stress reduction techniques. Your doctor will also start you on a multivitamin. Your adrenal glands need vitamin C, B vitamins, calcium, magnesium, zinc, selenium, copper, sodium, and manganese. Adaptogenic herbs are also very beneficial, such as ashwagandha, *Panax ginseng, Rhodiola rosea,* and *Cordyceps sinensis.* Calming herbs, such as chamomile and lemon balm, can be very beneficial. If you are not improving, your healthcare provider may discontinue the adaptogenic herbs and begin you on adrenal extracts after approximately six months.

If your cortisol level is still low after another three to six months, then your doctor may add licorice root to your therapy regimen. Licorice root decreases the amount of hydrocortisone that is broken down by the liver, which reduces the demand on the adrenals to produce more cortisol. Licorice root can raise your blood pressure, so it should not be taken if you have hypertension. If you develop high blood pressure while taking it, then discontinue its use.

If your DHEA level is low, your healthcare provider can prescribe you

DHEA. It is important that you also take the herbal therapies, otherwise when your DHEA is measured again the level may be even lower despite your taking it. If all other therapies fail and your cortisol level is still low, then your healthcare provider may prescribe Cortef to take for six months. It is the therapy of last resort. Your doctor will keep you on adrenal extract or adaptogenic herbs while you are taking the Cortef so that you have a therapy available for your body to use when it comes time to wean yourself off Cortef, which can take at least a month.

Usually, it takes six months of constant stress or more for adrenal fatigue to settle in. However, once you start treatment for your exhausted adrenals, it takes one to two years for your glands to heal completely.

There are other things you can do to help treat adrenal fatigue. Restful sleep (sleeping until 9 AM), resolving a stressful situation, lying down during a break from work, going to bed early (around 9 PM), and avoiding eating fruit in the morning can all help. Clearly, trying these options before things get out of hand is a good idea. Improving adrenal fatigue with these therapies can shorten healing time.

Many men who have adrenal fatigue also have a thyroid that isn't functioning to its full potential (hypothyroidism). It is important to always work on fixing the adrenal glands before thyroid medication is instituted; otherwise, the symptoms of adrenal fatigue may be made worse.

Adrenal fatigue is a phenomenon that can dramatically affect your health and can be reversed with proper treatment. Lifestyle changes, good nutrition, dietary supplements, and stress reduction techniques have all proven to be effective.

CORTISOL AND STRESS

When you are stressed, cortisol levels rise. As stress decreases, levels come back down. However, in today's world, a lot of people are stressed a lot of the time. Overbooking is an issue with almost everyone. If you have too many tasks on your plate or you multitask all the time, your body will remain in a state of constant stress. One study showed that as many as 75 percent to 90 percent of visits to primary care doctors are related to stress. In fact, chronic stress has been shown to contribute to accelerated aging and premature death. Another study revealed that chronic stress accelerated the aging process and was associated with shortened telomeres.

The most important thing you can do to get rid of your stress is to gain control of your time. Learn to say "no" kindly. Know how much work and responsibility you can take on without feeling overwhelmed, and do not take on more than you can handle. It is also useful to practice some relaxing techniques that you can turn to in times of stress. Running a hot bath, drinking a cup of coffee or tea, listening to your favorite song, or curling up with a good book are all effective ways to reduce stress. Figure out what works for you and turn to it if you feel your stress levels rising.

Carl Sandberg, a famous American poet, once wrote:

> *Time is the coin of your life. It is the only coin you have,*
> *and only you can determine how it will be spent.*
> *Be careful lest you let other people spend it for you.*

Stress can be harnessed to fuel success and achievement. However, if your stress is to the point of "distress," then that is a problem. Magnesium, potassium, B vitamins, vitamin C, zinc, carbohydrates, and other nutrients are used up when you are stressed.

Your brain is one of the body parts that is most affected by stress. When you are stressed and your cortisol levels increase, your body produces more free radicals. This damages your neurons and decreases your ability to think and remember things. When this happens, your body's ability to change short-term memories into long-term memories is affected. Your ability to recall and retrieve information is also impacted by stress. High levels of cortisol are associated with deterioration of the hippocampus, the part of your brain that processes memory.

OTHER SIGNS OF STRESS

By this point, you have learned that stress greatly affects cortisol levels, causing them to elevate. Elevated cortisol levels can have many negative consequences. (See page 31.) Over the years, I have compiled a list of common signs of stress, which can be divided into four categories.

Behavioral symptoms may be seen in the way you act. Some behavioral symptoms include bossiness, compulsive eating or gum chewing, excessive smoking, grinding your teeth at night, alcohol abuse, and an inability to focus on and complete tasks.

Cognitive symptoms are those that affect the way you think. If you are stressed, you may experience constant worry, forgetfulness, memory loss, or a lack of creativity. Additionally, you may have difficulty making decisions, lose your sense of humor, or have thoughts of running away.

Emotional symptoms affect your mood and feelings. If you're stressed, you may find that you are easily upset. Additionally, you may experience a range of emotions, including anger, boredom, edginess, loneliness, nervousness, anxiety, and unhappiness. Finally, people who are stressed commonly feel like they are under pressure, and they often feel powerless to change anything.

Lastly, there are some **physical symptoms** of stress that can affect your body. These include back pain, dizziness, headaches, a racing heart, restlessness, indigestion, stomachaches, tiredness, sweaty palms, a stiff neck or shoulders, ringing in the ears, and difficulty sleeping.

If you find that you are experiencing any of these symptoms, it would be a good idea to try and lower your levels of stress. (Some suggestions for how you can do this are on page 44.) You will greatly benefit in the long run.

In addition to stress, cortisol levels also increase with depression, infections, inadequate sleep, inflammation, hypoglycemia (low blood sugar), pain, and toxic exposure.

■ Signs and Symptoms of Elevated Cortisol

- ❏ Binge eating
- ❏ Compromised immune system
- ❏ Confusion
- ❏ Fatigue
- ❏ Favors the development of leaky gut syndrome
- ❏ Impaired hepatic conversion of T4 to T3 (see thyroid section on page 61)
- ❏ Increased blood pressure
- ❏ Increased blood sugar
- ❏ Increased cholesterol
- ❏ Increased insulin and insulin resistance
- ❏ Increased risk of developing osteoporosis/osteopenia
- ❏ Increased susceptibility to bruising
- ❏ Increased susceptibility to infections
- ❏ Increased triglycerides
- ❏ Irritability
- ❏ Low energy
- ❏ Night sweats
- ❏ Shakiness between meals
- ❏ Sleep disturbances
- ❏ Sugar cravings
- ❏ Thinning skin
- ❏ Weakened muscles

■ Effects of Stress on the Immune System

- Decreased release of antibodies

- Increased inflammatory cytokines

- Inhibition of the proliferation of T cells

- Inhibition of the release of certain interleukins

- Latent virus activation

- Shift from Th1 to Th2 cytokine expression

Lowering your cortisol level, if it is elevated, is very important. Stress-reduction techniques and a multivitamin are key components to start you on your way to normalizing your cortisol level. As previously mentioned, adaptogenic herbs such as ashwagandha, *Panax ginseng, Rhodiola rosea, Cordyceps sinensis,* and *Ginkgo biloba* are very beneficial if you feel stressed, and calming herbs such as lemon balm and chamomile are helpful if you feel wired. If cortisol is high in the evening, then add phosphatidylserine (300 mg) which may be taken at any point during the day.

ADPTOGENIC HERBS FOR CHRONIC STRESS

Plant adaptogens are compounds that increase the ability of an organism to adapt to environmental factors and to avoid damage from these factors. The beneficial effects of multi-dose administration of adaptogens are mainly associated with the hypothalamic-pituitary-adrenal (HPA) axis, a part of the stress-system that is believed to play a primary role in the reactions of the body to repeated stress and adaptation.

Each of these herbal therapies has a different mechanism of action. The best adaptogens to treat chronic stress are ashwagandha, bacopa, cordyceps, and holy basil. Each of these herbal therapies has a different mechanism of action.

ASHWAGANDHA

Grown in India, Pakistan, and Sri Lanka, ashwagandha (*Withania somnifera*) is part of the nightshade family. The roots of ashwagandha are known to improve resistance to emotional and physical stress and to benefit the body in other ways, as well. Ashwagandha is available in capsule form or can be made into a tea. Recommended capsule dosages range from 500 to

2,000 milligrams daily. Recommended dosages of dried root prepared in tea range from 3 to 4 grams daily.

■ Functions of Ashwagandha in Your Body

- Activates the immune system
- Enhances endurance and strength
- Has antibacterial properties
- Has anti-inflammatory properties
- Has cytotoxic (cell-killing) and tumor-sensitizing actions

- Helps preserve adrenal function
- Helps with stress reduction
- Increases libido and sexual performance
- Increases muscle mass
- Is an antioxidant
- Lowers cholesterol
- Protects the liver

■ Therapeutic Benefits of Ashwagandha

- Anxiety
- Asthma
- Back pain
- Constipation
- Coronary heart disease
- Depression
- Fever
- Fibromyalgia
- Hiccups
- Hypocholesterolemia (high cholesterol)
- Hypothyroidism (underactive thyroid)
- Infection (antibacterial and antifungal)

- Inflammation
- Insomnia
- Insulin resistance
- Memory loss
- Mood swings
- Osteoarthritis
- Stress
- Tardive dyskinesia
- Weakness

■ Possible Side Effects and Contraindications of Ashwagandha

- Diarrhea
- Nausea
- Vomiting

BACOPA

Bacopa (*Bacopa monnieri*) has been used for many years in Ayurvedic medicine to revitalize nerves, brain cells, and the mind. Bacopa helps to strengthen the adrenal glands and purify the blood. Studies have shown that it may have beneficial effects for anxiety and mental fatigue. Dosage: 200 to 400 mg a day and should be taken with food.

■ Functions of Bacopa in Your Body

- Enhances acetylcholine
- Improves transmission of nerve impulses
- Increases the body's utilization of nitric oxide
- Is effective against H. Pylori
- Regulates dopamine production
- Regulates serotonin production

Bacopa can intensify the activity of thyroid-stimulating drugs or inhibit the effectiveness of thyroid-suppressant drugs. Bacopa can have a sedative effect, therefore use caution when combining it with other sedatives. Possible side effects can occur, particularly if taken on an empty stomach.

■ Possible Side Effects and Contraindications of Bacopa

- Bloated stomach
- Cramping
- Dry mouth
- Fatigue
- Nausea

A study revealed that bacopa was able to provide protective effects against multitasking. In addition, bacopa improved both cognitive performance and mood in 1 to 2 hours. The recommended dosage ranges from 320 to 650 mg.

■ Therapeutic Benefits of Bacopa

- ADHD
- Allergies
- Alzheimer's disease
- Anxiety
- Diabetic neuropathy
- Epilepsy

- Hypertension
- Improves focus
- Irritable bowel syndrome (IBS)
- Pain relief
- Protects the kidneys
- Stress

CORDYCEPS

Cordyceps (*Cordyceps sinsensis* and *Cordyceps militaris*) is a fungus that has long been used in traditional Chinese and Tibetan medicine. Because natural cordyceps is difficult to obtain and is expensive when available, most supplements are made with cordyceps that has been created in a laboratory (Cordyceps CS-4).

Cordyceps is nutritionally rich, containing various types of essential amino acids; vitamins B_1, B_2, B_{12}, and K; carbohydrates; and trace elements. Studies have indicated that cordyceps can boost energy and oxygen during exercise, improve heart health, and combat inflammation, cancer, diabetes, and aging.

The recommended dosage is 400 milligrams twice a day. Be sure to use a pharmaceutical grade product, as some lower-grade products have been found to contain lead.

■ Functions of Cordyceps in Your Body

- Has antibacterial properties
- Has anti-cancer properties
- Has anti-inflammatory properties
- Has antimicrobial properties
- Has antioxidant properties
- Improves cardiac output

- Improves heart rhythm
- Improves kidney function
- Improves lung capacity
- Increases energy levels
- Lowers blood sugar levels
- Lowers cholesterol levels

- Lowers fibrinogen (a clotting factor)
- Modulates the immune system
- Protects the nervous system
- Provides adrenal support for stress

■ Therapeutic Benefits of Cordyceps

- Asthma
- Bronchitis
- Cancer
- Cardiac arrhythmia (irregular heartbeat)
- Chronic kidney disease (use only a healthcare provider's direction)
- Congestive heart failure
- Coughs
- Diabetes
- Hepatic cirrhosis
- Hepatitis B
- High cholesterol
- Infection
- Sexual dysfunction
- Stress due to adrenal fatigue

■ Possible Side Effects and Contraindications of Cordyceps

- Can cause problems when taken with medications such as prednisolone, as well as with antiviral or diabetic medications
- Discontinue use two weeks before surgery
- Do not take cordyceps if you are allergic to mold, have an autoimmune disease, or are pregnant or breastfeeding
- May increase the risk of bleeding if you have a bleeding disorder or are taking medications that change bleeding time

HOLY BASIL

Holy basil (*Ocimum sanctum*) is also known as tulsi. It is an aromatic plant that has been used for thousands of years. It is considered by many practitioners to be the best of the adaptogens in Ayurvedic medicine.

Holy basil can be used as a raw fresh whole herb. As dried leaves the dose is 300 to 600 mg a day for prevention, and 600 to 1,800 mg in divided doses as a therapy. There are no reported toxicities or adverse effects and no interactions have been described.

■ Functions of Holy Basil in Your Body

- Acts as a diuretic
- Enhances the immune system
- Has anti-anxiety properties
- Helps protect against heavy metal toxicity
- Helps protect from gamma radiation
- Helps protect from radioactive iodine
- Helps with fatigue
- Improves blood pressure if it is too low
- Is an adaptogen
- Is an antibacterial, antifungal, antimalarial, anti-parasitic, and antiviral agent

- Is an anticoagulant
- Is an antidepressant
- Is an anti-inflammatory
- Is an antioxidant
- Is an aphrodisiac
- Lowers blood sugar
- Lowers cholesterol
- Lowers temperature if elevated
- Promotes cognitive enhancement
- Protects against cancer
- Protects the liver
- Reduces stress from noise

■ Therapeutic Benefits of Holy Basil

- Allergy
- Anti-androgenic
- Anxiety
- Arthritis
- Asthma
- Back pain
- Bioremediation of contaminated air and soil
- Cardiopathy
- Cataracts

- Cough
- Diabetes
- Diarrhea and dysentery
- Earache
- Eye diseases
- Fever
- Food and herb preservation
- GI tract disorders
- Hand sanitizer
- Hiccups

- Indigestion
- Infertility
- Insect, snake, and scorpion bites
- Ischemic heart disease
- Leukoderma (loss of pigmentation of the skin)
- Malaria
- Metabolic syndrome
- Mouthwash

- Pain control
- Ringworm
- Skin disorders
- Stroke
- Ulcers
- Urinary diseases
- Vomiting
- Water treatment
- Wound healing

■ Possible Side Effects and Contraindications of Holy Basil

Avoid using Holy basil if you are allergic or sensitive to members of the *Lamiaceae* (mint) family. Possible side effects to this herb are an upset stomach. Also use with caution if you have low blood sugar.

ADPTOGENIC HERBS FOR ACUTE STRESS

A single-dose application of an adaptogen is important in situations that require a rapid response to tension or a stressful situation. In this case, the effects of the adaptogen are associated with another part of the stress system, namely, the sympatho-adrenal-system (SAS), which provides a rapid-response mechanism mainly to control the acute reaction of the organism to a stressor. SAS-mediated stimulating effects of single doses of adaptogens have been associated with *Rhodiola rosea, Schisandra chinensis,* and *Eleutherococcus senticosus.* Furthermore, these adaptogens effectively increase mental performance and physical working capacity in humans.

Eleutherococcus (or simply Eleuthero), Rhodiola, and Schisandra have all been found to be effective. Rhodiola is the most active of the three plant adaptogens, producing within thirty minutes of administration a stimulating effect that continues for at least 4 to 6 hours. In addition, a combination of herbal therapies can be beneficial for acute stress. Each of these herbal therapies has a different mechanism of action.

ELEUTHERO

Eleuthero (*Eleutherococcus senticosus*)—a species of shrub found in China, Korea, Japan, and Russia—has long been used by natural healers to increase energy, enhance endurance, and boost immunity. For many years, it was called Siberian ginseng because its effects are similar to those of ginseng. That name is now rarely used in the United States because it implies that the herb is part of the Panax genus (like American and Asian ginseng), while it actually belongs to the genus Eleutherococcus. Regardless of the controversy over its name, this herb is used to treat a variety of ailments. The recommended dosage ranges from 500 to 1,000 milligrams daily. Eleuthero can be taken for three months, followed by three to four weeks off.

■ Functions of Eleuthero in Your Body

- Acts as a stimulant
- Acts as an adaptogen to help your body manage stress
- Acts as an anti-inflammatory
- Acts as an antioxidant
- Aids the immune system by increasing T-cell and natural killer cell activity
- Improves endurance
- Improves learning ability
- Increases mental awareness
- Increases physical performance and stamina
- Increases tolerance to excessive heat, noise, and workload
- Promotes healing

■ Therapeutic Benefits of Eleuthero

- Anxiety
- Chronic fatigue
- Common cold and flu
- Crohn's Disease
- Diabetes
- Fibromyalgia
- Herpes simplex type 2 infection
- Hypercholesterolemia (high cholesterol)
- Increases physical work capacity in males
- Inflammation
- Insomnia

- Joint pain
- Kidney disease
- Liver disease
- Memory loss

- Osteoarthritis
- Rheumatoid arthritis
- Stress

■ Possible Side Effects and Contraindications of Eleuthero

- Can also interact with drugs taken to treat an autoimmune disease, drugs taken after organ transplant, steroids, digoxin, lithium, and sedatives (especially barbiturates).

- Can lower blood sugar levels. If you are being treated for insulin resistance or diabetes, monitor your blood sugar levels often to make sure they don't get too low.

- Do not use if you have a history of heart disease, hypertension, sleep apnea, narcolepsy, mania, or schizophrenia, or if you are pregnant or breastfeeding.

- Has a blood-thinning effect. If you have a bleeding disorder or are taking a medication or supplement that may thin your blood, do not take this herb. If you are planning to have surgery, discontinue this herbal therapy two weeks before the procedure.

RHODIOLA

Rhodiola (*Rhodiola rosea*) grows in cold, mountainous regions of Asia and Eastern Europe. Traditionally, this herb—which is known to contain more than 140 active ingredients—is used to treat anxiety, fatigue, and depression. It belongs to a group of plants known as adaptogens, which can help your body adapt to physical and environmental stress. Active compounds like rosoavin are able to balance the stress hormone cortisol.

The recommended dosage ranges from 200 to 600 milligrams a day in divided doses of standardized 3-percent rosavin and 1-percent salidroside.

■ Functions of Rhodiola in Your Body

- Decreases depression
- Has antibacterial properties

- Improves mental function
- Improves physical performance

- Is an adaptogen that helps the body manage stress

- Is an anti-inflammatory

- Is an antioxidant

- Lowers blood sugar levels

- Protective of the heart

- Protective of the liver

- Protective of the nervous system

- Reduces anxiety

■ Therapeutic Benefits of Rhodiola

- Altitude sickness

- Anxiety

- Cognitive problems

- Depression

- Insulin resistance/diabetes

- Nicotine dependence

- Physical and mental stress

■ Possible Side Effects and Contraindications of Rhodiola

Rhodiola decreases the possible liver side effects associated with the chemotherapeutic drug Adriamycin. It has a synergistic effect with cyclo-phosphamide's anti-tumor effect and decreases the risk of developing liver toxicity. The side effects of Rhodiola use are usually mild if any occur. At high doses, they may include:

- Allergic symptoms

- Fatigue

- Insomnia

- Irritability

SCHISANDRA

Schisandra is also an effective adaptogenic herb that has immediate action. It has many functions in the body.

■ Functions of Schisandra in Your Body

- Acts as an antibacterial

- Decreases allergies

- Decreases anxiety

- Decreases spasms in the GI tract

- Enhances exercise endurance

- Generates alterations in the basal levels of nitric oxide

- Has anti-cancer activity

- Helps protect the heart

- Helps to control blood sugar

- Improves bone mineralization

- Improves cortisol levels, positively affects the blood cells, vessels, and central nervous system

- Improves erectile dysfunction

- Increases endurance and accuracy of movement

- Increases mental performance

- Increases working capacity

- Inhibits leukotriene formation

- Is a platelet-activating factor antagonist

- Is an anti-inflammatory

- Is an antioxidant

- Is kidney protective

- Is liver protective

- Is neuroprotective

- Lowers cholesterol

- Modulates neurotransmitter function

- Promotes weight loss

- Regulates immune system

■ Therapeutic Benefits of Schisandra

- Acute gastrointestinal diseases

- Alcoholism

- Allergic dermatitis

- Asthenia (lack of energy)

- Asthma

- Cardiovascular disorders

- Chronic cough

- Chronic sinusitis

- Depression

- Dyspnea

- Hypotension (low blood pressure)

- Impaired visual function

- Influenza

- Insomnia

- Irritability

- Liver dysfunction

- Mediterranean fever

- Memory maintenance

- Neuritis

- Neurosis

- Night sweats

- Otitis (ear infection)

- Otosclerosis (inherited disorder)

- Palpitations

- Pneumonia
- Stomach and duodenal ulcers

- Stress
- Wound healing

■ Possible Side Effects of Contraindications of Schisandra

If you are on any medication, contact your healthcare provider before beginning this herb since it may interact with drugs that are metabolized by the CYP3A4 (an important enzyme that oxidizes toxins and drugs) system. In addition, there may be an elevation of serum levels of drugs that are P-glycoprotein substrates (play a role in transporting drugs to organs in the body) when taken with this herb. *Schisandra* may produce mild gastrointestinal discomfort.

COMBINATION THERAPIES FOR ACUTE STRESS

A study showed that *Panax ginseng, Rhodiola rosea,* and *Schisandra chinensis* were adaptogens that had numerous functions, and their effects were found to be very different in patients, depending on circumstances such as age, gender, environment, diet. Consequently, make sure your healthcare provider or pharmacist works with you on herbal therapies that you are thinking about taking.

■ Nutrients Associated with Increased Adrenal Function

- B vitamins
- Calcium
- Copper
- Magnesium
- Manganese
- Omega-3-fatty acids, such as fish oil

- Phosphatidylserine
- Selenium
- Sodium
- Vitamin C
- Zinc

As discussed previously, all the hormones in your body work together like a symphony. In order for you to have good health, they have to be balanced and at optimal levels. When cortisol levels are elevated, the thyroid gland is directly affected. The thyroid hormone produced may become stored, or bound, in the body, and therefore it may be unavailable for your body to use.

■ Factors Regulated by Neurotransmitters

- Appetite
- Memory
- Mood
- Muscle growth and repair

- Sexual interest
- Sleep
- Thirst
- Weigh

The simplest way to stop your cortisol levels from increasing is to better manage your stress. However, as you get older, this becomes more difficult because your ability to bounce back after a stressful event is reduced. Each event takes a deeper and more lasting toll on your body. Premature aging and many age-related disorders can begin with excessive stress.

Of course, abnormal levels of cortisol can occur at any age, but there are certainly different factors that can affect stress levels. One such factor is your job. Some jobs create more stress than others.

■ Most Stressful Occupations According to the National Institutes of Health

- Construction worker
- Farm worker
- Foreman/supervisor
- House painter
- Laboratory technician

- Machine operator
- Midlevel manager
- Secretary
- Waiter or waitress

The jobs on the list have one thing in common: a lack of control. Remember, you may not be able to control the things that are stressing you, but you can control how you respond to the stress. In other words, the key is not to avoid stress, but to change your perspective and how you respond to stress.

■ Optimal Cortisol Levels Helps to Prevent or Improve These Diseases

- Alzheimer's disease and other forms of cognitive decline
- Anorexia nervosa
- Anxiety disorders
- Chronic fatigue syndrome
- Coronary heart disease
- Decreases risk of infection
- Depression
- Fibromyalgia
- Impotence
- Infertility
- Insulin resistance/diabetes
- Irritable bowel syndrome (IBS)
- Multiple sclerosis
- Osteopenia/osteoporosis
- Panic disorders
- Post-traumatic stress disorder (PTSD)
- Rheumatoid arthritis
- Sleep disorders

As you have seen in this section, stress affects most every function in the body and is involved in almost all disease processes. A small amount of stress helps your body heal. Too much stress harms your body. Stress reduction techniques are a key component to healing. Prayer, meditation, tai chi (a Chinese form of martial arts), yoga, chi gong (a form of body and mind therapy), breathing exercises and techniques, exercise (mild exercise if you have adrenal fatigue), music, acupuncture, and dancing have all been shown to be therapeutic.

In order to be healthy, you have to be physically healthy, emotionally healthy, and spiritually healthy. All these areas of your life must be optimally functioning in order for you to enjoy a stress-free existence.

DIHYDROTESTOSTERONE (DHT)

Dihydrotestosterone (DHT) is the most potent naturally occurring androgen. It is three times more potent than testosterone. It is synthesized from the conversion of testosterone via the enzyme 5-alpha reductase. Testosterone conversion accounts for at least 70 percent of plasma DHT in the male. Androstenedione is also a precursor for DHT. DHT cannot be aromatized to estrogens. DHT has a growth promoting effect on prostate cells that is greater than that of testosterone. It is 2.4 to 10 times greater.

■ Functions of DHT in Your Body

- Formation of male sex-specific characteristics
- Responsible for the development of male genitalia and prostate
- If you have a low DHT level, you may have decreased sexual function and libido as well as decreased muscle tone.

■ Sources of DHT

- 5-alpha-reductase converts testosterone to dihydrotestosterone (DHT).
- Androstenedione is also a pro-hormone for DHT.

■ Signs and Symptoms of Elevated DHT Levels in Your Body

- ❏ Hirsutism (extra hair growth)
- ❏ Male pattern baldness
- ❏ BPH (Benign prostatic hyperplasia), prostate gland enlargement
- ❏ Decreasing DHT production, 5ARIs can decrease the size of the prostate
- ❏ High DHT levels stimulate the androgen receptors to produce greater amounts of PSA.

- ❏ DHT interacts with extracellular tissues to elevate prostate cancer cell mobility.
- ❏ DHT binds to androgen receptors in prostate cell nuclei and promotes proliferation of the cells
- ❏ High DHT levels have been shown to enhance early atherosclerosis (buildup of fats, cholesterol in arterial walls).

■ Cause of Elevated DHT

The only known cause of elevated DHT is being over prescribed 5-alpha reductase inhibitors. Replacement of this hormone is not suggested at this time.

■ Therapeutic Benefits

- Sexual dysfunction

PREGNENOLONE

Pregnenolone is synthesized from cholesterol. It makes estrogen, progesterone, testosterone, DHEA, and cortisol. Pregnenolone levels decline with age. By the age of seventy-five, most patients have 65 percent less pregnenolone than they did at age thirty-five. In addition to making the previously listed hormones, pregnenolone performs a variety of other functions in the body.

■ Functions of Pregnenolone in Your Body

- Blocks production of acid-forming compounds

- Enhances acetylcholine (chemical in the brain that acts as a neurostransmitter) neurotransmission

- Enhances nerve transmission and memory

- Helps repair nerve damage

- Improves energy (both physically and mentally)

- Improves sleep

- Increases resistance to stress

- Modulates NMDA receptors (regulate pain control, learning, memory, and alertness)

- Modulates the neurotransmitter GABA (calming neurotransmitter)

- Promotes mood elevation

- Reduces pain and inflammation

- Regulates the balance between excitation and inhibition in the nervous system

- Stimulates formation of new brain cells

■ Signs and Symptoms of Pregnenolone Deficiency

- ❏ Arthritis

- ❏ Depression

- ❏ Fatigue

- ❏ Insomnia

- ❏ Lack of focus

- ❏ Memory decline

■ Causes of Pregnenolone Deficiency

- Aging

- Eating too much saturated fat and trans fat

- Having a severe illness or dealing with prolonged stress

- Hypothyroidism

- Low cholesterol levels (total cholesterol needs to be 140 ng/dL to make pregnenolone)
- Pituitary dysfunction

At any age, pregnenolone will make more cortisol and less of the other hormones to help the body deal with stress.

■ Recommended Daily Dosage of Pregnenolone

Your blood level of pregnenolone must be at least 50 ng/dL to help maintain memory. Work with your healthcare provider to determine what dose of pregnenolone is best for you. A common starting dose is 10 mg. It is usually taken in the morning.

■ Possible Side Effects and Contraindications of Pregnenolone

It is contraindicated in patients with a history of hormonally related cancers, such as breast and prostate. Three percent of breast cancers occur in males. Supplementation may decrease the seizure threshold in people with a history of seizure disorder. Therefore, commonly lower doses of pregnenolone are used in these individuals.

■ Signs and Symptoms of Excess Pregnenolone

- ❑ Acne
- ❑ Anger
- ❑ Anxiety
- ❑ Drowsiness
- ❑ Fluid retention
- ❑ Headache
- ❑ Heart racing/palpitations
- ❑ Insomnia due to overstimulation
- ❑ Irritability
- ❑ Muscle aches

■ Causes of Excess Pregnenolone

- Pituitary tumor
- Taking too high a dose of pregnenolone

■ Therapeutic Benefits of Pregnenolone

- Allergic reactions
- Ankylosing spondylitis

- Arthritis
- Cannabis intoxication
- Depression
- Fatigue
- Insomnia
- Lupus
- Memory loss

- Moodiness
- Multiple sclerosis
- Psoriasis
- Rheumatoid arthritis
- Scleroderma
- Spinal cord injuries

INSULIN

Insulin is the hormone responsible for the regulation of blood sugar. Insulin is produced in the body with peak functioning of the pancreas along with optimal balancing of other hormones. Perfect insulin levels are a key to the best health possible. Insulin levels that are too high or too low can cause symptoms and increase the risk of developing several diseases.

■ Functions of Insulin

- Affects glycogen (storage form of glucose) metabolism by stimulation of glycogen synthesis
- Aids other nutrients to get inside cells
- Counters the actions of adrenaline and cortisol in the body
- Has an anti-inflammatory effect on endothelial cells (cells that release substances to control vascular relaxation/contraction and blood clotting) and macrophages
- Helps convert blood sugar into triglycerides
- Helps the body repair itself
- Increases expression of some lipogenic enzymes (converts glucose to triglycerides)
- Keeps blood glucose levels from rising too high
- Partially regulates protein turnover rate

- Plays a major role in the production of serotonin

- Stimulates the development of muscle (but at high levels it turns off the production of muscle and increases the production of fat)

- Suppresses reactive oxygen species (ROS)

Have your healthcare provider measure your fasting level, which is a blood study. Fasting serum insulin is used as an index of insulin sensitivity and resistance. The optimal fasting insulin level is 6 uIU/mL. Insulin levels that are too low or too high signify that insulin is not working optimally in your body. Commonly your doctor will measure your fasting blood sugar (FBS) and maybe also your hemoglobin A1c. Your hemoglobin A1c test tells you your average level of blood sugar over the past two to three months. It's also called HbA1c, glycated hemoglobin test, and glycohemoglobin. It is rare unless you are seeing a practitioner that specializes in Precision/Anti-Aging medicine that you would have your fasting insulin level measured. Make sure you request this test from your doctor.

■ Signs and Symptoms of Insulin Deficiency

- ❏ Blurred vision
- ❏ Bone loss
- ❏ Confusion
- ❏ Depression
- ❏ Dizziness
- ❏ Fainting
- ❏ Fatigue
- ❏ Hunger
- ❏ Hypoglycemia
- ❏ Insomnia
- ❏ Insulin resistance
- ❏ Loss of consciousness (late stage)
- ❏ Palpitations
- ❏ Seizures (late stage)
- ❏ Sweating

■ Causes of Insulin Deficiency

- Eliminating carbohydrates from the diet

- Hypopituitarism (a disorder in which your pituitary gland doesn't produce enough hormones)

- Insulin resistance/diabetes

- Not eating enough

- Over-exercising without sufficient food and nutritional support

- Pancreatic diseases such as chronic pancreatitis, cancer of the pancreas, and cystic fibrosis

When you eat complex carbohydrates and simple sugars, your insulin levels climb. If you eat too much sugar, your body produces more and more insulin until the insulin level is elevated and it does not work as effectively as it should. The medical term for this is insulin resistance.

■ Conditions Associated With Excess Insulin Production

- Acceleration of aging

- Acne

- Acromegaly

- Asthma

- Cushing's syndrome

- Depression and mood swings

- Heart disease

- Heartburn

- Hypercholesterolemia (high plasma cholesterol levels)

- Hypertension

- Hypertriglyceridemia (triglyceride levels are elevated)

- Increased risk of developing cancer

- Infertility

- Insomnia

- Insulin resistance/diabetes

- Irritable bowel syndrome

- Metabolic syndrome

- Migraine headaches

- Osteopenia/osteoporosis

- Weight gain

Insulin is part of the hormonal symphony in your body, so when it is not performing optimally, all the other hormones are affected. Your body will attempt to compensate for insulin's decreased effects by producing more and more insulin. This can result in high insulin levels all the time, which can cause the cells in your adrenal glands, called theca cells, to turn on an enzyme called 17, 20-lyase. It may also promote further insulin resistance. In fact, prolonged levels of high insulin can lead to diabetes.

Furthermore, most major processes that lead to hardening of the arteries are caused by the overproduction of insulin.

When you eat simple sugars and consume caffeine to help with fatigue, not only will your adrenal glands suffer, but this will contribute to an elevated level of insulin in your body. Additionally, this causes your body to produce gas and you may experience bloating. Water is pulled into your colon from the bloodstream to respond to the high sugar load, which can lead to loose stools. Moreover, you may develop gluten sensitivity from overeating carbohydrates.

There are many habits that can elevate insulin besides eating a diet high in simple sugars. Having a lot of stress, which causes your cortisol levels to be abnormal, will have a negative impact on insulin production. The following list contains lifestyle choices that raise insulin, as per Dr. Diana Schwarzbein, an endocrinologist and author of *The Schwarzbein Principle* and *The Schwarzbein Principle II*.

■ Causes of Excess Insulin Production

- Cigarette smoking
- Consuming soft drinks
- Eating a low-fat diet
- Eating trans fats (partially hydrogenated or hydrogenated)
- Elevated DHEA levels
- Excessive alcohol consumption
- Excessive caffeine intake
- Excessive or unnecessary thyroid hormone replacement
- Increased testosterone levels
- Lack of exercise
- Poor sleep hygiene
- Skipping meals
- Some over-the-counter cold medications (any that contain caffeine)
- Some prescription medications (these are the most common)
  - Beta-blockers
  - Levodopa
  - Some medications for depression and psychosis
  - Steroids
  - Thiazide diuretics
- Stress
- Taking diet pills
- Taking thyroid hormone replacement while not eating enough
- Use of artificial sweeteners

- Use of natural stimulants
- Use of recreational stimulants
- Yo-yo dieting

Elevated insulin levels can be lowered by eating a balanced diet of carbohydrates, proteins, and fats. The right amount of exercise (three or four times a week) can help to normalize insulin levels. Changing medications, quitting smoking, discontinuing stimulants, and decreasing or stopping caffeine consumption can also be beneficial. In addition, there are nutrients that can help insulin work more effectively in the body. Alpha lipoic acid, chromium, and vitamin D all do just this. However, these supplements can be very powerful, so if you are already taking a drug that lowers your blood sugar, you may need less medication with the use of these products.

Make sure you monitor your blood sugar closely. Alpha lipoic acid has even been shown to prevent and treat diabetic neuropathy, a condition in which the body's nerves become damaged due to diabetes. (See "Insulin Resistance" below for further information.)

■ Therapeutic Benefits of Optimal Insulin Levels

- Helps to normalize weight
- Memory maintenance
- Prevention and treatment of insulin resistance and diabetes
- Prevention of coronary heart disease
- Prevention of hypertension
- Prevention of osteoporosis/ osteopenia
- Prevention of some cancers

INSULIN RESISTANCE

Insulin resistance is evident when cells do not properly absorb glucose, the body's preferred source of fuel, resulting in a buildup in the blood. If left untreated, insulin resistance may lead to prediabetes, a condition in which glucose levels are higher than normal but not high enough to be considered diabetes. Insulin resistance occurs when insulin is present but does not work as effectively in the body as it should. Consequently, levels start to rise to help the body compensate for less than effective insulin function.

More than 80 percent of the adult population in the United States has blood glucose levels that are too high. If a patient has a fasting blood sugar (FBS) that is high-normal (over 85 mg/dL), the risk of the person dying of cardiovascular disease (heart disease) is increased by 40 percent. Furthermore, having a FBS that is high-normal increases the patient's risk of vascular death. Insulin also plays a profound role in cognitive function. High-normal levels of FBS may account for a decrease in the volume of the hippocampus and amygdala of 6 to 10 percent. Consequently, insulin resistance is a risk factor for cognitive decline. Also, the "Honolulu-Asia Aging Study" showed that the effect of hyperinsulinemia (high insulin levels) on the risk of dementia was independent of diabetes and blood glucose. Therefore, growing evidence supports the concept that insulin resistance is important in the pathogenesis of cognitive impairment and neurodegeneration.

■ Sign and Symptoms of Insulin Resistance

❑ Fuzzy brain

❑ Infertility (possible role in the impairment of glycolysis in sperm cells)

❑ Irritability

❑ Loose bowel movements alternating with constipation

❑ Water retention

❑ Weight gain

■ Causes of Insulin Resistance

Insulin resistance has many possible causes. Here are some reasons why individuals with insulin resistance are not able to effectively use insulin.

- Abuse of alcohol
- Decreased testosterone
- Eating processed foods
- Elevated DHEA levels
- Excessive caffeine intake
- Excessive dieting
- Genetic susceptibility
- Hypothyroidism
- Increased stress
- Insomnia
- Lack of exercise
- Use of nicotine

Conventional therapies for insulin resistance involve exercise and a diet centered on consumption of foods with low glycemic index numbers.

If an individual is overweight, then weight reduction is very beneficial. If these methods are not successful, then nutrients and medications such as Glucophage may be added.

Precision/Anti-Aging Medicine has many therapies to improve and sometimes even reverse insulin resistance. The first one is exercise. Lack of exercise is a risk factor for the development of insulin resistance and diabetes in susceptible individuals. Exercising four days a week for an hour a day has been shown to be beneficial. Eating foods that are low on the glycemic index (GI) is important. The GI ranks carbohydrate-containing foods on a scale from 0 to 100 according to the speed with which they enter the bloodstream and raise glucose levels. Foods high on the list increase blood sugar and cause insulin to rise.

One study showed that insulin secretion was lower in people who were on a low glycemic index program for only two weeks. The glycemic index is affected by the size of the particles into which the food breaks down. Therefore, the more the processed the food or the longer it is cooked, the higher its glycemic index. The best carbohydrates that curb insulin are broccoli, lentils, and chickpeas. In addition, the fat content of a food influences its glycemic index ranking. Good fats (monounsaturated and polyunsaturated) slow down sugar absorption and therefore lower the glycemic index number.

The right balance of saturated to polyunsaturated to monounsaturated fats is important both for the prevention and treatment of insulin resistance and diabetes. Likewise, a high-fiber diet is crucial. Soluble fiber has been shown to lower insulin levels. Furthermore, getting enough protein in the diet decreases the absorption of sugars and consequently decreases your glycemic load. Weight loss has been shown to be helpful as well. Moreover, getting a good night's sleep has been shown to be beneficial. If you do not sleep at least six and a half hours a night, then insulin levels may rise and lead to insulin resistance.

There are also many nutritional supplements and botanical nutrients that have clinical trials supporting their use in insulin resistance.

SUPPLEMENTS TO TREAT INSULIN RESISTANCE

Supplements with an asterisk (*) can have a blood-thinning action.

Supplements	Dosage	Considerations
Alpha lipoic acid	100 mg to 400 mg daily	Alpha lipoic acid improves blood sugar levels, so diabetics may be able to take less medication. Alpha lipoic acid also slows the development of diabetic neuropathy. Consult your healthcare provider if you are considering taking more than 500 mg in a day. Larger doses can negatively impact thyroid functioning.
Arginine	1,000 to 5,000 mg once a day	Do not take if you have kidney disease, liver disease, or herpes except under a doctor's supervision. Arginine can interact with some medications. Consult with your healthcare provider before beginning this therapy.
Asian ginseng*	50 to 200 mg of extract standardized to 4 percent ginsenosides twice a day	Always take with food. Use with caution if you have high blood pressure. Do not use if you are taking a blood thinner or if you have a hormonally related cancer such as breast or prostate.
B-complex vitamins	50 mg twice a day	I suggest taking a multivitamin along with your B-complex vitamins.
Berberine*	Start with 200 mg twice a day (You may go up to 500 mg three times a day)	It should be taken with a meal to be absorbed most effectively and to also help prevent gas and stomach upset.
Bergamot	800 mg once or twice a day	It also blocks the rate-limiting step in cholesterol production. If you are on a cholesterol lowering medication, have your healthcare provider measure your cholesterol after three months. You may need a lower dose of the drug.
Carnitine*	2,000 to 3,000 mg once a day	Have your healthcare provider measure your TMAO levels before starting long-term supplementation with carnitine.
Carnosine	2,000 mg once a day	Check with your doctor before starting carnosine therapy if you have diabetes, hypertension, kidney disease, or liver damage. Too much carnosine can result in hyperactivity.

Supplements	Dosage	Considerations
Chromium	300 to 1,000 mcg once a day as chromium picolinate	Combining with the protein picolinate allows your body to absorb chromium more efficiently. However, some chromium picolinate supplements contain more chromium than necessary. Ask your healthcare provider for a recommendation on chromium consumption.
Coenzyme Q10*	30 to 200 mg daily	If you are on blood-thinning medications, speak to your healthcare provider before using CoQ10. Since some medications can cause a deficiency of this nutrient, speak to your healthcare provider to determine if you might need a larger dose.
Copper	2 to 3 mg once a day	Your copper-to-zinc ratio is very important for your health. Also, do not take copper supplement cupric oxide, which has a very low bioavailability.
Cysteine	500 mg once a day as n-acetylcysteine, or NAC	When taking NAC supplements, also take extra vitamin C, copper, and zinc.
D-ribose	15,000 mg three times a day	D-ribose can lower blood sugar levels, so check with your healthcare provider before taking this supplement with any diabetes medication, especially insulin.
EPA/DHA (fish oil)*	1,000 to 2,000 mg once a day	Choose a source that contains vitamin E to prevent oxidation.
Fenugreek*	50 mg of seed powder twice a day, or 2 to 4.5 ml of 1:2 liquid extract twice a day	Avoid fenugreek if you are allergic to chickpeas, peanuts, green peas, or soybeans. Fenugreek has mild blood-thinning effects. If you have a bleeding disorder or are taking a medication or supplement that may thin your blood, do not take this herb. Fenugreek may also negatively impact thyroid functioning.
Fiber, soluble	Suggested daily intake is 25 grams for women and 38 grams for men (Try to get most of your fiber from whole foods)	Choose a fiber supplement with no added sugar, and take with several glasses of water to prevent side effects.
Ginkgo biloba*	120 mg once daily	Do not use with blood-thinning medications or supplements.

Supplements	Dosage	Considerations
Green coffee bean extract	400 mg a day	Because green coffee contains caffeine, you should avoid taking this supplement if you are sensitive to caffeine.
Gymnema sylvestre	400 to 600 mg a day of an extract that contains 24 percent gymnemic acid	Stop taking this supplement two weeks before surgery, as it can interfere with blood sugar control during and after surgical procedures. At high doses, gymnema can cause gastric irritation or liver toxicity.
Inositol	2,000 to 4,000 mg once a day	Doses larger than 200 mg should be taken only under physician supervision.
Magnesium	400 to 800 mg once a day	Consult your healthcare provider for dosage if you have kidney disease. Discontinue use and see your doctor if you experience abdominal pain. Take a lower dose if it causes diarrhea.
Manganese	2 to 5 mg once a day	Use with caution if you have gallbladder or liver disease.
Olive leaf extract*	500 mg to 750 mg a day containing 20 mg of oleuropein per capsule	Olive leaf extracts can interact with many prescription medications, and may increase the effects of blood thinners. Consult your healthcare provider before using olive leaf extract if you are taking any medication.
Quercetin*	300 mg three times a day	For best results, take with bromelain and vitamin C. Do not use with blood-thinning medications or supplements.
Selenium	200 mcg once a day	Do not exceed 200 mcg a day without consulting your healthcare provider.
Taurine	1,000 to 1,500 mg once a day	Take between meals. Discontinue use if you suddenly have feelings of chest or throat tightness or if you break out in hives. Do not take with aspirin. Have your healthcare provider measure levels before starting taurine therapy.
Vanadium*	50 mcg once a day	Do not take more than 50 mcg a day without a doctor's supervision. Do not use if you are taking blood-thinning medications or supplements.

Supplements	Dosage	Considerations
Vitamin B6 (pyridoxine)	75 mg twice a day	Do not take more than 500 mg a day. If you are taking L-dopa for Parkinson's disease, do not take B6 without first consulting your doctor. High doses can deplete your body of other vitamins in the B complex, so take a B-complex vitamin twice a day.
Vitamin B7 (biotin)	8 to 10 mg once a day	Large doses of biotin can deplete your body of other vitamins in the B complex, so take B-complex vitamins twice a day. Biotin can also negatively impact thyroid function.
Vitamin B12 (cobalamin)	500 to 1,500 mcg twice a day	High doses can deplete your body of other vitamins in the B complex, so take with a B-complex vitamin twice a day.
Vitamin C	500 to 1,500 mg twice a day	Do not take high doses if you are prone to kidney stones or gout. High doses can also cause diarrhea.
Vitamin D3	Have your blood levels measured by your healthcare provider, who will determine proper dosage	You can become vitamin D toxic. Therefore, have your healthcare provider measure your levels to determine the perfect dose for you.
Vitamin E*	400 to 800 IU once a day	Take mixed tocopherols, the more active type of vitamin E. Consult your healthcare provider first if you are taking a blood thinner.
Zinc	20 to 50 mg once a day as zinc picolinate or zinc citrate	Your copper-to-zinc ratio is very important to your health. If you are taking zinc and iron supplements, take one in the morning and one in the evening. (Taking them together reduces the efficiency of both.)

Many people in the United States and the remainder of the world have insulin resistance. The great news is that there are many therapies with proven clinical trials that have been shown to be effective in helping insulin to work more effectively in the body.

If insulin resistance occurs long enough, you can develop diabetes, which is discussed in Part II of this book. (See page 52.)

THYROID HORMONE

Your thyroid gland is your body regulator. Therefore, an imbalance of your thyroid hormone can affect every metabolic function in your body. Consequently, your thyroid gland has a lot of important functions.

■ Functions of the Thyroid Gland and Thyroid Hormone in Your Body

- Affects tissue repair and development

- Aides in the function of mitochondria (energy makers of your cells)

- Assists in the digestion process

- Controls hormone excretion and balance of other hormones

- Controls oxygen utilization

- Modulates blood flow

- Modulates carbohydrate, protein, and fat metabolism

- Modulates muscle and nerve action

- Modulates sexual function

- Regulates energy and heat production

- Regulates growth

- Regulates vitamin usage

- Stimulates protein synthesis

TYPES OF THYROID HORMONE

As you age it becomes more common for thyroid problems to occur. There are a few different types of thyroid hormones and a stimulating hormone that your body produces. They are:

- Thyroid stimulating hormone (TSH), which is made in your pituitary gland located in your brain

- Diiodothyronine (T2) is produced from T3 and from reverse T3

- Triiodothyronine (T3), which is made in other tissues

- Thyroxine (T4), which is made in your thyroid gland

T4 is 80 percent of the thyroid gland's production. Most of T4 is converted into T3 in your liver or kidneys. T3 is five times more active than T4. T4 can also be converted into reverse T3, which is an inactive (stored) form. Additionally, T2 increases the metabolic rate of your muscles and fat tissues and its levels decrease with advancing age.

Thyroid Hormone and Iodine

Iodine, a chemical element, is particularly important when considering thyroid function. Iodine is an antibacterial, anticancer, antiparasitic, antiviral, and mucolytic agent.

Iodine is needed to maintain healthy breast tissue and nerve function, and it protects against toxic effects from radioactive material. According to the World Health Organization, up to 72 percent of the world's population is affected by an iodine deficiency disorder.

Causes of Iodine Deficiency

- Diet high in pasta and breads with contain bromide (bromide binds to the iodine receptors)

- Diet low in salt

- Diet without ocean fish or sea vegetables, such as seaweed

- Fluoride use (inhibits iodine binding)

- Ground depleted of iodine

- Medications that contain fluoride or bromide

- Sucralose (contains chlorinated table sugar)

- Vegan and vegetarian diets

Contrary to the foods that interfere with iodine, there are plenty of foods that are useful sources of iodine.

Food Sources of Iodine

- Beef
- Beef liver
- Bread, whole wheat
- Butter
- Cheese, cheddar
- Cheese, cottage

- Clams
- Cream
- Eggs
- Green peppers
- Haddock
- Halibut
- Lamb

- Lettuce
- Milk
- Oysters
- Peanuts
- Pineapple
- Pork
- Raisins

- Salmon
- Sardines (canned)
- Shrimp
- Spinach
- Tuna (canned)

Be aware, however, that if you intake too much iodine you can get acne. Excess iodine intake can also cause thyroiditis, an inflammation of the thyroid gland that results in overproduction of the thyroid hormone. Your healthcare practitioner can measure your iodine levels with a urine test.

If you need iodine replacement, it will most likely contain iodine and iodide. Iodine replacement comes in both a liquid and tablet form. About one third of people treated for low thyroid function will need to have a lower dose of thyroid medication when the iodine deficiency is corrected.

Your body can produce too little or too much thyroid hormone. Too little thyroid hormone production is called hypothyroidism. Excessive thyroid hormone production is termed hyperthyroidism. See inset on page 66 for an extensive discussion of these disorders.

Decreased production of T3 can cause high cholesterol, because low levels of T3 cause less cholesterol to be removed from your blood. This causes an increase in bad cholesterol. Individuals who have low thyroid levels have cholesterol levels that are 10 to 50 percent higher than people with normal thyroid function.

Inadequate thyroid function can stimulate CYP3A4, a part of the P450 system in the liver, which can cause an increase in production of 16-hydroxy estrone, which can increase your risk of developing prostate cancer.

Decreased thyroid hormone levels can be caused by a variety of factors. Sometimes, a deficiency of certain minerals or vitamins can lead to low T4 production.

◼ Nutritional Deficiencies That Can Cause a Decrease in T4 Production

- Copper
- Zinc
- Vitamins A, B_2, B_3, B_6, and C

◼ T4 to T3 Conversion

Your body also needs to be able to convert T4 to T3. T3 is the more active form of thyroid hormone. This conversion requires an enzyme called 5'diodinase.

The inability to convert T4 to T3 will lead to symptoms of thyroid hormone loss. As discussed earlier, T4 also sometimes converts into reverse T3, which can also lead to symptoms of thyroid loss.

◼ Effects of Decreased T3 (or Increased Reverse T3)

- Aging
- Chronic fatigue
- Diabetes
- Fasting
- Fibromyalgia
- IL-6, TNF-alpha, IFN-2 (immune system factors)

- Increased catecholamines (epinephrine and norepinephrine)
- Increased free radicals
- Infections
- Prolonged illness
- Stress
- Toxic metal exposure
- Yo-yo dieting

As mentioned, the conversion of T4 to T3 cannot take place without 5'diodinase, an enzyme. There are many factors that can affect your body's production of this important enzyme.

Reverse T3

Reverse T3 is a measurement of inactive thyroid function. Reverse T3 has only 1 percent of the activity T3 does. It is an antagonist of T3, which means that the higher your reverse T3 level is, the lower your T3 level will be. T3 and reverse T3 bind to the same receptor sites, so they cannot both occupy these sites at the same time. This situation occurs due to a malfunction of the metabolism of T4. When your reverse T3 is high this is a medical syndrome now called "reverse T3 dominance."

The most common reason that reverse T3 levels become elevated is stress. When you are stressed, your cortisol levels rise. If you stay stressed all the time your cortisol levels will stay elevated (see page 28). This phenomenon can cause your body to produce more reverse T3.

Risk Factors and Causes of Reverse T3 Dominance

- Diet low in fruit
- Diet low in green vegetables
- High estrogen levels are found more and more commonly in men
- High intake of red meat
- High-fat diet
- History of abuse
- Immune dysfunction
- Lack of exercise from an early age on
- Mitochondrial dysfunction
- Naturally red hair

When you have a high reverse T3 level, you can have any or all of the symptoms of hypothyroidism (low thyroid function) that have been discussed in this section. The most common symptom that I see in my practice in patients who have high reverse T3 levels is weight gain. It is very difficult to lose weight and keep it off if your reverse T3 levels remain elevated. Unfortunately, weight gain is also very discouraging. It may make dealing with other problems seem more difficult.

Additionally, when your reverse T3 level is high your body temperature goes down. This slows the action of many enzymes in your body, which can lead to a syndrome called "multiple enzyme dysfunction."

Causes of Multiple Enzyme Dysfunction

- Exposure to environmental estrogens or estrogen disruptors (PCBs, weed killers, plastics, detergents, household cleaners, and tin can liners)
- Liver dysfunction
- Long-term exposure to dioxin (a class of toxic chemicals)
- Poor estrogen metabolism
- Prenatal exposure to high levels of estrogen

Consequently, it is very important to have your reverse T3 levels measured. Some scientists believe that the best indicator of thyroid function is the ratio between T3 and reverse T3 since this ratio measures the tissue levels of thyroid hormone.

High levels of reverse T3 can be treated in several ways. Taking the nutrients that aid the conversion of T4 to T3 is very beneficial. Selenium, zinc, vitamins B_6 and B_{12}, iron, vitamin D, and iodine, if levels are low, have all been found to be helpful. If you are taking T4 medication, discontinuing it can also increase T3 and lower reverse T3 levels. Always consult your healthcare provider before discontinuing any drug. In addition, taking T3 as a prescription will also increase T3 levels and decrease reverse T3. Furthermore, if you have elevated cortisol levels, lowering them to normal will also diminish your reverse T3.

■ Factors That Affect 5'diodinase Production

- Cadmium, mercury, or lead toxicity
- Chronic illness
- Decreased kidney or liver function
- Elevated cortisol
- Herbicides, pesticides
- High carbohydrate diet
- Inadequate protein intake
- Polycyclic aromatic hydrocarbons
- Selenium deficiency
- Starvation
- Stress

There are other factors besides insufficient 5'diodinase levels that can lead to an inability to convert T4 to T3 effectively.

■ Additional Factors That Cause an Inability to Convert T4 to T3

- Aging
- Alpha-lipoic acid (600 mg a day or more)
- Calcium excess
- Certain medications (these are the most common)
  - Beta-blockers
  - Chemotherapy
  - Lithium
  - Phenytoin
  - Theophylline
- Copper excess
- Deficiencies in the following nutrients
  - Iodine
  - Iron
  - Selenium
  - Vitamins A, B_2, B_6, and B_{12}
  - Zinc
- Diabetes
- Dietary factors

- Cruciferous vegetables (too many)
- Excessive alcohol intake
- Low carbohydrate diet
- Low fat diet
- Low protein diet
- Soy
- Walnuts (excessive intake)
- Dioxins
- Fluoride
- Lead
- Inadequate production of adrenal hormones (DHEA, cortisol)
- Mercury
- PCBs
- Pesticides
- Phthalates (chemicals added to plastics)
- Radiation
- Stress
- Surgery

Moreover, iron deficiency and physical inactivity impair your body's response to T3. These factors will also cause you to have symptoms of hypothyroidism.

On the contrary, there are factors that will increase the conversion of T4 to T3 if there is not enough T3 being made by your body.

■ Factors That Increase the Conversion of T4 to T3*

- Ashwagandha
- Glucagon
- Growth hormone
- High protein diet
- Insulin
- Iodine
- Iron
- Melatonin
- Potassium
- Selenium
- Testosterone
- Tyrosine
- Vitamins A, B$_2$, and E
- Zinc

You may notice that some of the same things that decrease the conversion of T4 to T3 also increase it. This is due to the fact that it is important to have the right amount of these nutrients, herbs, and hormones in your body. Too much or too little will affect thyroid production and, subsequently, function.

Signs and Symptoms of Hypothyroidism

Early diagnosis of hypothyroidism isn't always easy. Most people with an underactive thyroid aren't aware that they have this condition. They may suffer a number of symptoms without recognizing that the symptoms are thyroid-related or that there may be no symptoms early on in the disease process. Often times, the physician may minimize or misdiagnose the symptoms. The signs and symptoms of hypothyroidism normally progress slowly, over months or years, and quite often they may be confused with other disorders. The following are signs and symptoms of hypothyroidism:

- Acne
- Agitation/irritability
- Allergies
- Anxiety/panic attacks
- Arrhythmias (irregular heart rhythm)
- Bladder and kidney infections
- Blepharospasm (eye twitching) is more common
- Carpel tunnel syndrome
- Cholesterol levels that are high (hypercholesterole-mia)
- Cognitive decline
- Cold hands and feet
- Cold intolerance
- Congestive heart failure
- Constipation
- Coronary heart disease/acute myocardial infarction (heart attack)
- Decreased cardiac output
- Decreased sexual interest
- Delayed deep tendon reflexes
- Deposition of mucin (glycoprotein) in connective tissues
- Depression
- Dizziness/vertigo
- Down turned mouth
- Drooping eyelids
- Dull facial expression
- Ear canal that is dry, scaly, and may itch
- Ear wax build-up in the ear canal (cerumen)
- Easy bruising
- Eating disorders
- Elbow that are rough and bumpy (keratosis)
- Endometriosis
- Erectile dysfunction
- "Fat pads" above the clavicles
- Fatigue
- Fibrocystic breast disease
- Fluid retention
- Gallstones
- Hair loss in the front and back of the head
- Hair loss in varying amounts from legs, axilla, and arms
- Hair that is sparse, coarse, and dry
- Headaches including migraine headaches
- High cortisol levels
- High C-reactive protein (CRP)
- Horse, husky voice
- High homocysteine levels (hyperhomocystein-emia)

- High insulin levels (hyperinsulinemia)
- Hypertension
- Hypoglycemia (low blood sugar)
- Impaired kidney function
- Inability to concentrate
- Increased appetite
- Increased risk of developing asthma
- Increased risk of developing bipolar disorder
- Increased risk of developing schizoid or affective psychoses
- Infertility
- Insomnia
- Iron deficiency anemia
- Joint stiffness (arthralgias)
- Loss of eyelashes or eyelashes that are not as thick
- Loss of one-third of the eyebrows
- Low amplitude theta and delta brain waves.
- Low blood pressure
- Low body temperature
- Menstrual cycle pain
- Menstrual irregularities including abnormally heavy bleeding
- Mild elevation of liver enzymes
- Miscarriage
- Morning stiffness
- Muscle and joint pain
- Muscle craps
- Muscle weakness
- Muscular pain
- Nails that are brittle, easily broken, ridged, striated, thickened nails
- Need to get up and urinate in the middle of the night (nocturia)
- Nutritional imbalances
- Osteoporosis (bone loss)
- Abnormal sensation of feeling burning, tingling, and itching (paresthesia)
- Poor circulation
- Poor night vision
- Premenstrual syndrome (PMS)
- Puffy face
- Reduced heart rate
- Ringing in the ears (tinnitus)
- Rough, dry skin
- Shortness of breath
- Sleep apnea
- Slow movements
- Slow speech
- Swollen eyelids
- Swollen legs, feet, hands, and abdomen
- Tendency to develop allergies
- Vitamin B12 deficiency
- Weight gain
- Yellowish skin discoloration due to the inability to convert beta carotene into vitamin A

There are some conditions that may be or may not be signs and symptoms of hypothyroidism, such as growth hormone deficiency in children, retrograde uterus, vitiligo, skin cancer, dry eyes, TMJ, and teeth clenching. If you suffer from any one or a number of these health issues, and no root cause has not been found to alleviate the problem, perhaps it's time to consider looking at how well your thyroid is functioning.

OTHER TESTS OF THYROID FUNCTION

Besides blood studies, your doctor can do some other tests to look at thyroid function.

- **Thyroid scan.** A thyroid scan is a common test that is done to determine if you have a thyroid nodule (a lump that arises on the thyroid gland) and if the nodule is hot or cold. If you have a goiter (enlargement of the thyroid gland), its size can be measured by a thyroid scan. If you have had thyroid cancer, then a thyroid scan can be used after surgery to see if you have a reoccurrence of cancer. A thyroid scan is also used to determine if you have thyroid tissue located outside of the neck. The scan is done by giving a radioisotope (like radioactive iodine) and letting the thyroid gland (or thyroid tissue outside of the thyroid) take up the isotope.

- **Thyroid ultrasound.** A thyroid ultrasound is another method of testing thyroid function and assessing thyroid nodules. With this study, sound waves are used to tell if a thyroid nodule is solid or a cyst. However, this test will not tell your doctor if the nodule is cancerous or benign (non-cancerous). If your healthcare practitioner needs more information, you may be sent for a biopsy of your thyroid gland.

- **Basal body temperature.** Some people will have normal or even optimal levels of thyroid hormone but still will have symptoms of hypothyroidism. For these individuals it is important to get a basal body temperature. A basal body temperature is the temperature underneath your arm taken before you get out of bed in the morning for ten minutes. You take your temperature for three consecutive days. If you are menstruating, then take your temperature during your menstrual cycle.

- **Thyroid binding globulin (TBG).** Thyroid binding globulin (TBG) can also be measured. Thyroxine-binding globulin is one of three major transport proteins, which are primarily responsible for binding to and transporting thyroid hormones to the necessary tissues. The other two serum transport proteins include transthyretin and human serum albumin. Thyroid binding globulin is produced by the liver and is affected by illness, liver disease, and some medications. Sometimes estrogens can raise TBG so this is another test that you doctor may order.

- **Thyroid Releasing Hormone (TRH).** Your healthcare provide r may also order a thyroid releasing hormone (TRH) level which is a hormone made in the hypothalamus that stimulates the release of thyroid stimulating hormone (TSH) and prolactin from the pituitary. TRH expression is activated by energy demanding situations, such as cold and exercise, and it is inhibited by negative energy balance situations, such as fasting, inflammation, or chronic stress.

Some individuals have an autoimmune process where their body is literally trying to attack its own thyroid gland and the body produces a normal amount of thyroid hormone or not enough thyroid hormone. This is called Hashimoto's thyroiditis. If you have Hashimoto's thyroiditis, your test results will reveal that your thyroid antibody levels are high. Your thyroid antibodies can also be increased if you have a special kind of hyperthyroidism (over production of thyroid hormones) called Graves' disease.

MELATONIN

Melatonin is a hormone produced in the pineal gland, retina, GI tract, and white blood cells, and is associated with sleep. In addition, there are melatonin receptors expressed all over the body—for example, in the intestines, fat tissue, kidneys, liver, lungs, adrenals, and other organs. The amount of melatonin the body produces decreases as one ages and depends on the activity of an enzyme called serotonin-N-acetyltransferase (NAT). The body's production of NAT, on the other hand, depends on its storage of vitamin B_6. Melatonin has many functions in your body.

■ Functions of Melatonin in Your Body

- Acts as an antioxidant

- Aids the immune system

- Decreases cortisol levels that are elevated

- Decreases platelet stickiness (decreases the risk of heart disease)

- Dilates and contracts blood vessels

- Effects the release of sex hormones

- Helps balance the stress response

- Helps prevent cancer and treat some cancers

- Improves mood
- Improves sleep quality
- Inhibits the release of insulin from beta cells in the pancreas
- Inhibits the release of prolactin, follicle stimulating hormone (FSH) and luteinizing hormone (LH)
- Is cardioprotective
- Promotes healthy cholesterol levels

- Protects against GI reflux
- Protects skin cells against UV damage
- Regulates skin pigmentation
- Relieves jet lag
- Stimulates the parathyroid gland
- Stimulates the production of growth hormone

■ Signs and Symptoms of Melatonin Deficiency

- ❑ Anxiety
- ❑ Compromised immune system
- ❑ Early morning awakening
- ❑ Fatigue
- ❑ Heart disease
- ❑ Immunological disorders

- ❑ Increased risk of cancer
- ❑ Insomnia
- ❑ Interrupted sleep
- ❑ Seasonal affective disorder
- ❑ Stress

■ Causes of Melatonin Deficiency

There are many etiologies of melatonin deficiency. Perhaps the most common cause of melatonin deficiency in today's world is electromagnetic fields. Other causes include the following.

- Acetaminophen
- Alcohol abuse
- Aspirin/indomethacin/ ibuprofen
- Caffeine abuse

- High glycemic index foods
- Some medications
- Tobacco
- Vitamin B_{12} and B_6 deficiency

■ Therapeutic Benefits of Melatonin

The therapeutic benefits of melatonin are numerous. Melatonin is a hormone that does much more than regulate the sleep cycle.

Alzheimer's Disease. Some of the symptoms of low melatonin levels are also common to patients with Alzheimer's disease: disruption of the circadian rhythm of the body, mood changes, and delirium. One medical trial showed that melatonin levels in the CSF (cerebrospinal fluid) in patients over the age of eighty were one-half the level of younger, healthier individuals. Individuals in this study with Alzheimer's disease had even lower levels—only 20 percent of the amount observed in young healthy people. Fortunately, numerous studies have shown that supplementing with melatonin helps to protect against Alzheimer's disease. In addition, in animal and human trials a benefit in melatonin replacement in patients with early Alzheimer's disease was seen even before it was clinically evident. In fact, when melatonin was replaced early, the participants did not show pathological changes nor have symptoms of cognitive decline.

In addition, melatonin supplementation has been shown to decrease the damage caused by amyloid beta proteins, both of which increase the risk of developing Alzheimer's disease. Moreover, medical trials revealed that using melatonin in patients with Alzheimer's disease resulted in better sleep patterns, less sundowning, and slower progression of cognitive loss. Likewise, melatonin has also been shown to guard against the harmful effects of aluminum, which has been shown to cause oxidative changes in the brain that are similar to those seen in Alzheimer's disease.

Cancer. Many studies have shown that melatonin is an effective therapy for breast cancer as an adjunct to traditional care. It has also been shown to be effective in the prevention and reduction of some of the side effects of chemotherapy and radiation, including mouth ulcers, dry mouth, weight loss, nerve pain, weakness, and thrombocytopenia (low platelet count). Moreover, melatonin has been used as a therapy for other cancer forms, such as brain, lung, prostate, head and neck, and gastrointestinal cancers.

Cerebral Vascular Accident (CVA). If a person has a low melatonin level, they have an increased risk of developing a cerebral vascular accident (stroke). The odds rise more than 2 percent for every 1 pg/mL decline in melatonin. In fact, in individuals with a calcified pineal gland, the risk of developing a CVA is increased by 35 percent. Moreover, melatonin supplementation has been shown to shrink the size of an infarct area in a patient with acute CVA. This may be due to melatonin's ability to neutralize free-radical production.

Melatonin may also decrease the risk of CVA by significantly lowering cholesterol and decreasing blood pressure. Furthermore, melatonin supplementation in lab animals decreased the damage after stroke and decreased seizure occurrence. In addition, melatonin has been shown to increase plasticity of neurons after CVA. Likewise, in animal studies, melatonin reduced the damage caused by stroke by decreasing the activation of "protein-melting" enzymes. Melatonin has also been shown to tighten the blood-brain barrier, reduce tissue swelling, and prevent hemorrhagic transformation in animal trials with experimentally induced stroke.

Closed Head Injury (CHI)/Traumatic Brain Injury (TBI). Supplementation with melatonin has been shown to minimize the brain swelling and dysfunction that occurs after a closed head injury. Melatonin supplementation has also been shown to help protect the brain in the case of traumatic brain injury. Likewise, studies employing lab animals have shown that giving melatonin after a TBI had the following results: maintained the integrity of the blood-brain barrier, prevented dangerous brain swelling in the hours and days after injury, and shrank the size of the bruised and injured tissue. Melatonin, likewise, reduced the mortality rate after burst aneurysm in laboratory studies.

COVID-19. Melatonin is now being used as an adjuvant treatment for COVID-19, since it has been shown to limit virus-related diseases. It has also been demonstrated to be protective against acute lung injury and adult respiratory distress syndrome caused by viruses and other pathogens due to its anti-inflammatory and anti-oxidative effects. Unfortunately, Covid-19 tends to take a more severe course in individuals with chronic metabolic diseases such as obesity, diabetes mellitus, and hypertension. Since Covid-19 complications frequently involve severe inflammation and oxidative stress in this population, melatonin is being suggested as an add-on therapy for patients that are diabetic and overweight.

Gastrointestinal Diseases. The enterochromaffin cells (most common endocrine cells in the GI tract) of the gastrointestinal tract secrete 400 times as much melatonin as the pineal gland. Consequently, it is not surprising that numerous studies have found that melatonin plays an important role in GI functioning. As previously mentioned, melatonin is a powerful antioxidant that resists oxidative stress due to its capacity to directly scavenge reactive species, increase the activities of antioxidant enzymes, and stimulate the innate immune response through its direct and indirect actions. In the gastrointestinal tract, the activities of melatonin are mediated by melatonin receptors, serotonin, and cholecystokinin B receptors, as well as through receptor-independent processes.

Let us now examine the use of melatonin in several disease processes of the GI tract. The prevalence of gastroesophageal reflux disease (GERD) is increasing with individuals experiencing symptoms such as heartburn, regurgitation, dysphagia, coughing, hoarseness, or chest pain. Fortunately, melatonin has been shown to have inhibitory activities on gastric acid secretion and nitric oxide biosynthesis. Nitric oxide has an important role in transient lower esophageal sphincter relaxation which is a major cause of reflux in people with this disease process.

A study revealed that a combination of melatonin, L-tryptophan, vitamin B_6, folic acid, vitamin B_{12}, methionine, and betaine was beneficial for patients with GERD. In addition, the other components of the formula exhibit anti-inflammatory and analgesic effects. All patients that took the combination of nutrients and melatonin reported a complete regression of symptoms after forty days of treatment. However, only 65.7 percent of the omeprazole patients reported regression of symptoms in the same period. Numerous other studies have also revealed that melatonin has a role in the improvement of gastroesophageal reflux disease when used alone or in combination with the drug omeprazole.

In addition, melatonin can protect the GI mucosa from ulceration by its antioxidant action, stimulation of the immune system, limitation of gastric mucosal injury, and promotion of epithelial regeneration. Melatonin can also reduce the secretion of pepsin and hydrochloric acid and influence the activity of the myoelectric complexes of the gut via its action in the central nervous system. This hormone furthermore attenuates acute gastric lesions and accelerates ulcer healing via its interaction with melatonin receptors due to an enhancement of the gastric microcirculation.

Similarly, melatonin is a promising therapeutic agent for irritable bowel syndrome (IBS), with activities independent of its effects on sleep, anxiety, or depression due to its important role in gastrointestinal physiology. It regulates gastrointestinal motility, has local anti-inflammatory reaction, and moderates visceral sensation. Studies have consistently shown improvement in abdominal pain, some trials even revealed improvement in quality of life in these individuals. In fact, studies have regularly publicized that alteration of the circadian rhythm is associated with the development of digestive pathologies that are linked to dysmotility or changes in microbiota composition in irritable bowel syndrome and similar conditions.

Moreover, disruption of circadian physiology, due to sleep disturbance or shift work, may result in various gastrointestinal diseases, such as irritable bowel syndrome, gastroesophageal reflux disease, or peptic ulcer disease. In addition, circadian disruption accelerates aging, and promotes tumorigenesis in the liver and GI tract. Furthermore, identification of the role that melatonin plays in the regulation of circadian rhythm allows researchers and clinicians to approach gastrointestinal diseases from a chronobiological perspective. Recently, it has been postulated that disruption of circadian regulation may lead to obesity by shifting food intake schedules. Likewise, a study suggests that sensing of bacteria through toll-like receptor 4 (TLR4) and regulation of bacteria through altered goblet cells and antimicrobial peptides is involved in the anti-colitic effects of melatonin. Consequently, melatonin may have use in therapeutics for inflammatory bowel diseases such as Crohn's and ulcerative colitis.

Heart Health. Patients with coronary artery disease tend to have low nocturnal serum melatonin levels. In addition, patients who developed adverse effects post myocardial infarction (MI) were shown to have lower nocturnal melatonin levels than patients without adverse effects. Melatonin is cardioprotective due to its vasodilator actions and free radical-scavenging properties. It also inhibits oxidation of LDL-C. Likewise, melatonin has been shown to reduce hypoxia and prevent reoxygenation-induced damage in individuals with cardiac ischemia and ischemic stroke.

The "MARIA" study was a prospective, randomized, double-blind, placebo-controlled trial that used IV melatonin in patients following an acute MI (heart attack) that were having angioplasty. It decreased CRP and IL-6, two major markers of inflammation. Melatonin also attenuated tissue damage from reperfusion (restoring the flow of blood to organs or tissue), decreased V tach (ventricular tachycardia) and V fib (ventricular fibrillation) after reperfusion. It also reduced cellular and molecular damage from ischemia. Another study revealed that there is an inverse correlation between melatonin levels and CRP levels after acute MI (myocardial infarction), a heart attack. Moreover, melatonin has been shown to protect cardiac myocyte mitochondria after doxorubicin (used for chemotherapy) use.

Hypertension. Melatonin has been shown to decrease blood pressure in patients with hypertension. In fact, a study revealed that evening controlled-release melatonin, 2 mg for one month, significantly reduced nocturnal systolic blood pressure in patients with nocturnal hypertension.

Immune Builder. Melatonin has been shown to be a major regulator of the immune system. Consequently, disease states affecting a wide range of organ systems have been reported as benefiting from melatonin administration.

Insulin Regulation and Obesity. Melatonin is necessary for the proper synthesis, secretion, and action of insulin. In addition, melatonin acts by regulating GLUT4 expression via its G-protein-coupled membrane receptors, the phosphorylation of the insulin receptor, and its intracellular substrates that mobilize the insulin-signaling pathway. GLUT4 is the insulin-regulated glucose transporter found primarily in adipose tissues (fat tissue) and striated muscle (skeletal and cardiac). Furthermore, melatonin is responsible for the establishment of adequate energy balance by regulating energy flow and expenditure through the activation of brown adipose tissue and participating in the browning process of white adipose tissue. Likewise, melatonin is a powerful chronobiotic, meaning that it helps regulate the body's internal clock.

Consequently, the reduction in melatonin production that may occur with aging, shift work, or illuminated environments during the night commonly induces insulin resistance, glucose intolerance, sleep disturbance, and metabolic circadian changes that commonly lead to weight gain. A study using laboratory animals showed that melatonin supplementation daily at middle age decreased abdominal fat and lowered plasma insulin to youthful levels. A low melatonin level is a frequently overlooked cause for an individual's inability to lose weight effectively.

Longevity. Lab trials have shown that melatonin replacement increases SIRT1, which is a longevity protein. SIRT1 is also activated by caloric restriction.

Mild Cognitive Impairment. Mild cognitive impairment (MCI) is impairment that precedes actual dementia. In fact, 12 percent of people with MCI proceed to develop dementia each year. Studies have shown that people who supplemented with melatonin (3 to 24 mg daily) for 15 to 60 months did much better on cognitive tests.

Neurodegenerative Disorders. Studies have shown that low melatonin levels are associated with an increased risk of developing neurodegenerative diseases such as Alzheimer's disease, mild cognitive impairment, cerebral vascular disease (stroke), and traumatic brain injury.

Parkinson's Disease. Melatonin replacement has been shown to decrease the risk of developing Parkinson's disease. Moreover, animal trials have shown that melatonin can prevent and, to some extent, may even help reverse the motor and behavioral changes that are associated with this disease process.

In Parkinson's disease there is an accumulation of a protein called alpha-synuclein. Melatonin supplementation also attacks alpha-synuclein and makes it more available to be removed by the body. In addition, a lab study showed that melatonin can reverse the inflammatory changes that occur in Parkinson's disease. Moreover, an animal trial also showed that melatonin helps to restore the normal activity of a key enzyme that is involved in the synthesis of dopamine. Furthermore, in lab studies melatonin supplementation was shown to increase the survival of dopamine-producing cells. Consequently, more research needs to be done concerning melatonin's use in Parkinson's disease.

Preoperative Anxiety. When compared to a placebo, melatonin given as premedication (tablets or sublingually), can reduce preoperative anxiety in adults. In fact, melatonin may be equally as effective as the standard treatment with midazolam in reducing preoperative anxiety. The effect of melatonin on postoperative anxiety in adults is mixed but suggests an overall attenuation of the effect compared with preoperative anxiety.

Sleep Hygiene. Melatonin has long been known to be beneficial for sleep. Melatonin has been shown to synchronize the circadian rhythms and improve the onset, duration, and quality of sleep. The good news is that exogenous melatonin supplementation is well tolerated and has no obvious short- or long-term adverse effects when used in small doses to improve sleep hygiene.

■ Other Sources of Melatonin

The following are common foods that contain melatonin.

- Asparagus
- Barley
- Black olives/green olives
- Black tea/green tea
- Broccoli
- Brussels sprouts
- Corn
- Cucumber
- Mushrooms

- Oats
- Peanuts
- Pomegranate
- Red grapes
- Rice
- Strawberries
- Tart cherries
- Tomatoes
- Walnut

■ Possible Side Effects and Contraindications of Melatonin

Melatonin is an immune stimulator. Therefore, it should be used with caution in individuals that have an autoimmune disease, leukemia, or lymphoma, people who suffer from mental illness, and anyone taking steroids.

■ Signs and Symptoms of Excess Melatonin

- ❏ Abdominal pain
- ❏ Daytime sleepiness/fatigue
- ❏ Depression
- ❏ Headaches
- ❏ Hypotension (low blood pressure)

- ❏ Increase in cortisol, which can increase fat storage
- ❏ Intense dreaming/nightmares
- ❏ Suppression of serotonin, which increases carbohydrate cravings
- ❏ Transient dizziness

■ Causes of Excess Melatonin

The most common reason that people have elevated levels of melatonin is that they take doses that are too large, or they take melatonin and do not need it. Likewise, an individual may also have high levels of melatonin if they eat too many foods that contain melatonin. Some medications, such as desipramine, fluvoxamine, thorazine, and tranylcypromine, may raise melatonin levels, as can St. John's wort supplementation. Ingesting the herb *Vitex agnus-castus* (chaste tree) can also lead to elevated melatonin levels. If melatonin levels are high, serotonin levels tend to decline. Therefore, it is important to test your melatonin levels, by salivary testing, if you are taking more than one mg of melatonin at night.

■ Melatonin Dosing Schedules

Common dosages for males of melatonin are 1 to 3 mg. In addition, medical studies have also suggested that patients may need less melatonin for insomnia as they age. As previously mentioned, large doses of melatonin are used to treat cancer. Likewise, very large doses of melatonin are now being employed as co-therapies for COVID-19 under a healthcare provider's direction. If melatonin is going to be used long-term, measuring levels is suggested.

Melatonin is a wonderful hormone that has so many functions in the body aside from regulating sleep. As you have seen, it has been shown to be an effective therapy for many disease processes along with a beneficial way to build the immune system.

CONCLUSION

As you have seen in Part I of this book, there are many hormones produced by your body. Discussed were many of the most important ones. It is paramount that all your hormones are balanced, and stay balanced, for you to achieve and maintain optimal health throughout your life.

PART II

Ailments and Problems

INTRODUCTION

For many years, science has ignored the role that hormonal function plays in the relationship between a man and his body. Issues such as insomnia, sexual dysfunction, and anxiety may be related to hormonal levels. How well you maintain vision, memory, and mobility are also related to optimal hormonal function. Even your risk of heart disease and stroke can be connected, in part, to your hormones.

Recent research has brought about many new medications and treatments to decrease your risk factors for disease and to help you live a healthier and longer life. An example of this is Precision/Anti-Aging Medicine. It is not a complementary or alternative specialty. Precision Medicine is a specialty that looks at the metabolism of the body and how the body works. It takes into consideration that medical problems are highly individualized. The same symptoms in two different people may mean entirely different things.

Part II of this book takes a glimpse at the ailments and problems that can occur if your hormones are not balanced. One size does *not* fit all when it comes to your medical treatment. As always, working with a healthcare professional and pharmacist that are specially trained in this area is suggested. Additionally, when taking supplements, always consume them with a full glass of water and make sure you are taking pharmaceutical grade nutrients. Pharmaceutic grade supplements are ones that are bioavailable (are absorbed easily into your body) and are also free of toxins. There is no regulation on vitamins in some countries such as the United States. Consequently, it is always important to make sure you are taking vitamins and other nutrients that are pharmaceutical grade.

It is also imperative you note the following precautions, along with the considerations given for each supplement. The dosages listed are intended for adults without kidney or liver disease. If you have kidney or liver disease, you may need to take lower dosages of most supplements and you should consult your healthcare provider before embarking on any nutritional program. If you are taking *Coumadin* or any other blood thinner, your dosage of certain nutrients must be lower than what is suggested. Please ask your physician, pharmacist, or other healthcare provider for help determining the appropriate dosage. If you are having surgery, do not take any nutrients (except for the surgery pre- and post-operative protocol that your doctor gives you) for 10 days before and one week after your surgery date.

BENIGN PROSTATIC HYPERPLASIA (BPH)

Benign prostatic hyperplasia (BPH) refers to the nonmalignant growth or hyperplasia (enlargement) of prostate tissue and is a common cause of lower urinary tract symptoms in men. BPH occurs when both stromal and epithelial cells of the prostate in the transitional zone proliferate by processes that are thought to be influenced by inflammation and sex hormones, causing prostate enlargement. BPH does not usually occur before the age of 60. The incidence of benign prostatic hyperplasia increases with age until almost 90 percent of males in their 80s suffer from this disease.

■ Signs and Symptoms of BPH

An enlarged prostate gland can cause uncomfortable urinary symptoms.

- Burning on urination (can also be due to infection)

- Decreased force of urinary stream

- Frequency (having to urinate frequently)

- Hesitancy

- Incomplete bladder emptying (increased post-void residual urine volume)

- Nocturia (waking to urinate)

- Pain in upper thighs, lower back, or pelvis

- Post-void dribbling

- Straining or prolonged voiding

- Urgency (a strong and immediate need to urinate)

- Urinary frequency

Potential complications of BPH include the following: urinary tract infections, urolithiasis (formation of stony concretions in the bladder or urinary tract), urinary retention, renal insufficiency (decreased kidney function), and hematuria (blood in the urine).

Urology is moving away from the term benign prostatic hyperplasia to the term lower urinary tract symptomatology (LUTS) to describe voiding dysfunction in males. Therefore, you may see one or both of these terms describing BPH. Although LUTS is often associated with BPH, LUTS can also be due to unrelated syndromes, such as metabolic syndrome, heart failure, urinary tract infections, and diabetes.

Causes of BPH

The cause of BPH is not totally understood. It may be related to any of the following:

- Aging process

- Detrusor dysfunction (dysfunction of the detrusor muscle which can contract inappropriately) of the bladder neck

- DHT (dihydrotestosterone) increase inhibits prostate cell death and promotes cell proliferation (growth), so it increases the size of the prostate.

- Estrogens increase the number of DHT receptors in the prostate and inhibit androgen metabolism by interfering with hydroxylation which is a chemical process that introduces a hydroxyl group (-OH) into an organic compound.

- Genetic predisposition to BPH has been demonstrated in cohort studies, first-degree relatives in one study demonstrated a four-fold increase in the risk of BPH compared to control.

- Inflammation of the prostate with prostaglandin and leukotriene response

- Insulin resistance. Elevated insulin levels increase sympathetic nerve activity and also bind to insulin-like growth factor (IGF) receptors that stimulate prostate cell growth.

- Obesity, metabolic syndrome, and insulin resistance also increase inflammation systemically which is likewise associated with BPH.

- Partaking of seven or more alcoholic drinks per week is associated with worsening symptoms.

- Visceral fat that is excessive increases the circulation of estradiol (E2 estrogen) which further stimulates the growth of prostate cells by increasing DHT.

■ Therapies for BPH

Conventional Therapies

- Watchful waiting: If the symptoms are mild to moderate, then treatment is usually optional.

- Lifestyle modifications: Lifestyle modifications such as fluid restriction, frequent bladder emptying, and avoidance of bladder irritants are recommended for individuals with BPH of any severity.

▓ Medications

Alpha-1-adrenergic receptor-blocking agents

Possible side effects of alpha-1-adrenergic receptor blockers

- Asthenia
- Dizziness
- Ejaculatory problems
- Nasal congestion
- Orthostatic hypotension

- Intraoperative floppy iris syndrome. It is very important for a person to let their ophthalmologist (eye specialist) know if they are taking alpha-1-adrenergic receptor blockers if they are considering cataract surgery.

5-alpha-reductase inhibitors (5ARIs)

Possible side effects of 5ARIs

- Antimuscarinic agents
- Breast tenderness (rare)
- Combination of alpha-adrenergic receptor blocker and PDE-5 inhibitor
- Combination therapy with 5-alpha-reductase inhibitors and alpha blocker.
- Decreased libido
- Ejaculatory disorder
- Erectile dysfunction
- Phosphodiesterase type 5 inhibitor (PDE-5 inhibitors) may be a useful option for men with combined erectile dysfunction and others who want to mitigate the sexual adverse effects of other drugs for BPH.

■ Minimally Invasive Therapy

Transurethral microwave therapy (TUMT)

Risk of procedure

- Extended urethral catheterization may be needed
- Prolonged irritative voiding symptoms
- Urinary retention

Transurethral needle ablation (TUNA)

Risk of procedure

- Prolonged irritative symptoms
- Temporary urinary retention

Precision Medicine Therapies

- Promote prostate health
  - Decrease caffeine intake since it tends to tighten the bladder neck and make it harder to urinate
  - Decrease alcohol use since it tightens the bladder neck
  - Avoid prescription antihistamines and decongestant since they can cause the bladder neck to constrict. Use natural antihistamines, such as quercetin.
  - Avoid spicy and acidic foods
  - Decrease stress
  - Increase the frequency of sexual intercourse
  - Urinate before going to bed
  - Live in a warm climate in the winter

- Avoid things that can make BPH worse
  - Sympathetic stimulation increases tone of prostatic stroma, which causes constriction of the urethra and can also stimulate bladder spasm. Therefore, avoid the following herbal therapies: bitter orange, ephedra, country mallow, and yohimbe.
  - Anticholinergic stimulation can make urination more difficult by inhibiting bladder contraction and causing urinary retention.

Therefore, avoid the following herbal therapies: henbane, scopolia, jimson weed, and wild lettuce.

- Androgen hormonal stimulation (testosterone replacement) can accelerate the growth of the prostate if used in high doses or inappropriately.

- Testosterone

  - Testosterone deficiency may alter the structure of the lower urinary tract, such as urethral and bladder epithelial cells which may lead to BPH. Consequently, testosterone replacement, if testosterone levels are low, is suggested if you are a candidate for hormone replacement therapy. Conversely, too high a dose of testosterone can worsen BPH.

- Decrease conversion to dihydrotestosterone (DHT)

  - Decreasing conversion of testosterone to DHT may be helpful. This can be accomplished by your healthcare provider prescribing progesterone cream which is a natural inhibitor of 5-alpha reductase. It is compounded and made by a compounding pharmacy or by your doctor prescribing a 5-alpha-reductase inhibitor made by a pharmaceutical company.

- Normalize estrogen levels

  - Males make three different forms of estrogen which are important to help them maintain memory and bone structure. Estrogen in males is also neuroprotective, helps with lipid metabolism, and regulates gonadotropin feedback. The pituitary gonadotropins, luteinizing hormone (LH), and follicle-stimulating hormone (FSH), play a pivotal role in reproduction. In men, LH regulates the synthesis of androgens by the Leydig cells, whereas FSH promotes Sertoli cell function and therefore influences the making of sperm. However, elevated levels of estrogens in males increase their risk of BPH and also the risk of prostate cancer, heart disease, strokes, peripheral vascular disease, and carotid artery stenosis (carotid artery becomes blocked).

The following things can raise estrogen levels in males

- Alcohol abuse

- Aromatization of hormones

- Eat foods that increase estrogen level (see inset on page 87)

- Environmental estrogens
- Grapefruit
- High-dose vitamin E
- Liver disease
- Medications and OTC (over the counter) drugs
  - Abusive substances: alcohol, amphetamines, marijuana, cocaine
  - Antacids: omeprazole, cimetidine
  - Antibiotics: sulfa, tetracycline, penicillin, cefazolin, erythromycin, quinolone
- Antidepressants: fluoxetine, fluvoxamine, paroxetine, sertraline
- Anti-fungal agents
- Anti-psychotic medicines: Thorazine, haloperidol
- Cholesterol lowering drugs
- Heart and blood pressure medicines: propranolol, quinidine, amiodarone, coumadin, methyldopa
- Pain relievers: acetaminophen, NSAID, ASA, propoxyphene
- Obesity
- Zinc deficiency

The following are ways to lower estrogen levels in males

- Anastrozole and other aromatase inhibitors
- Chrysin (compounded it as a medication)
- Decrease alcohol intake
- Decrease dose of testosterone
- Decrease intake of estrogen containing foods (see inset on page 87)
- Eat foods that decrease estrogen (see inset on page 88)
- Eat organic foods and avoid environmental estrogens
- Grape seed extract
- High dose vitamin C (also increases testosterone production)
- Lose weight
- Maca
- Niacin
- Vitamin K
- Wild nettle root
- Zinc

Foods That Increase Estrogen

Vegetables

Artichoke	Cucumber	Potato (all kinds)
Asparagus	Eggplant	Pumpkin
Bamboo shoot	Garlic	Radish
Beet	Green beans	Seaweed
Brussels sprout	Lettuce	Shallot
Cabbage	Mustard greens	Spinach
Carrot	Okra	Tomato
Cauliflower	Onion	Turnip
Celery	Parsley	Yam
Chive	Pepper (red, green,	
Corn	yellow, orange)	

Fruits

Apple	Grapefruit	Pineapple
Apricot	Lemon	Plum
Banana	Muskmelon	Red grapes
Cherry	Orange	Strawberry
Date	Peach	Watermelon
Grape	Pear	

Cereals and Grains

Barley	Rice	Wheat (bran, flour,
Corn	Rye	whole)

Legumes (Beans)

Chickpea	Pea	Soybean
Kidney	Peanut	

Seeds and Nuts

Almond	Pecan	Sesame seed
Cashew	Pine nut	Sunflower seed
Coconut	Pistachio	Walnut

Most common oils

Coconut	Linseed (flaxseed)	Peanut
Corn	Olive	Rice bran

| Safflower | Soybean | Walnut |
| Sesame seed | Sunflower | Wheat germ |

Foods That Decrease Estrogen

Cruciferous vegetables

Broccoli	Cauliflower	Mushrooms: Baby
Bok choy	Collard greens	button, Cremini,
Brussels sprouts	Kale	Portabella, Shitake
Cabbage	Turnips	Rutabagas

Seeds that contain polyphenols

| Chia | Flax | Sesame |

Others

| Green tea | Pomegranates | |

- Dietary changes
  - Soy may be helpful for BPH since it inhibits 5-alpha-reductase. It is a low-potency estrogen and may block the estrogen receptor sites that the stronger estrogens use to increase DHT. In addition, one study found that patients that ate more garlic had less BPH. Moreover, high cereal intake increases the risk of developing BPH according to a study. If you eat a lot of cereal, consider decreasing your intake.

- Nutrients
  - Beta-sitosterol is a sterol found in various plants. It is usually extracted from South African star grass. Food sources are avocados, nuts, including almonds, macadamia, and peanuts. It is also contained in wheat germ and oils, such as olive, rice bran, sesame, corn, and canola. It has been shown to inhibit 5-alpha-reductase, which is an enzyme in the prostate that converts testosterone into dihydrotestosterone (DHT), which is growth promoting. Beta-sitosterol also has anti-inflammatory properties. In addition, it also has been shown to lower cholesterol. A common dose is 20 mg BID. Do not use plant sterols, including beta-sitosterol, if you have a rare autosomal recessive genetic disorder called phytosterolemia, which causes over-absorption of phytosterols. Few side effects have been reported.

- Lycopene is a carotenoid pigment found in tomatoes and other red or pink fruits, such as apricots, guavas, pink grapefruit, watermelon, and dark green leafy vegetables. It is an anti-inflammatory and also reduces oxidative stress therefore decreasing free radical production. Lycopene tends to concentrate in the prostate gland where it helps lower inflammation. Lycopene also has antiproliferative properties which prevent the abnormal growth of cells and may inhibit prostate enlargement. In cell studies, lycopene decreased prostate cell division. This nutrient also reduces the production of DHT, one of the hormones that cause the prostate to enlarge. Dose: 5 to 20 mg a day.

- Omega-3-fatty acids are beneficial for BPH. One study concluded that omega-3-fatty acids used in conjunction with tamsulocin and finasteride produced better clinical results than either alone. Another study found omega-3-fatty acids alone was helpful.

- Zinc is essential for a healthy prostate. High levels of zinc are needed for maintaining prostate health and function due to its role in apoptosis (cell death) and truncatin part of the Krebs cycle, which is the main energy producing cycle in the body. BPH has been associated with low zinc levels. Consider taking zinc. It is important to also remember to replace copper in a ratio of 10 to 15 mg of zinc to one mg of copper.

- Botanicals

  - Pygeum africanum has shown promise for the treatment of BPH. It is derived from the bark of the African cherry tree. Medical studies reveal that Pygeum bark extracts help control bladder overactivity and decrease prostate enlargement and nocturia (a medical condition in which you wake up during the night because you have to urinate).

  - Pumpkin seed oil (Cucurbita pepo) contains phytosterol which is a protective compound that may be responsible for reducing prostate enlargement and BPH symptoms. The German Research Activities on Natural Urologicals (GRANU) study was a randomized, partially blinded, placebo-controlled, parallel-group trial that investigated the efficacy of pumpkin seed in men with lower urinary tract symptoms, suggestive of benign prostatic hyperplasia. Overall, in men with BPH, 12 months of treatment with pumpkin seed led to a clinically relevant reduction in symptoms compared with placebo. Another study found it useful in the management of patients affected by LUTS-BPH for improving symptoms and quality of life.

- Rye grass pollen (Secale cereale) extract has been used for prostate conditions such as BPH in small studies. The most commonly used form is called Cernilton. The available evidence suggests that it is well tolerated. Larger studies need to be done.

- Saw palmetto (Serenoa repens) extract (SPE) is an extract from the ripe berries of the American dwarf palm and has been used as a therapeutic remedy for urinary dysfunction due to benign prostatic hyperplasia. SPE contains a complex mixture of free fatty acids and their esters, small quantities of phytosterols (for example, B-sitosterol), aliphatic alcohols, and various polyprenic compounds. Several studies have shown that SPE helps with the symptoms of BPH. Saw palmetto extract may exert a direct effect on the pharmacological receptors in the lower urinary tract, thereby improving urinary dysfunction in people with BPH and an overactive bladder. Dose: 150 mg twice a day. The following are possible side effects that are seen infrequently: altered hormonal activity, constipation, cramping, decreased sexual drive, diarrhea, headache, and nausea. Conversely, not all studies showed that saw palmetto was of benefit.

- Stinging nettle (Urtica dioica) is a perennial wild plant that originally came from Europe and Asia. Its name is derived from the tiny sharp hairs that encompass the plant and can irritate or sting the skin when the plant is touched. It has both anti-inflammatory and antioxidant activities. Only a few components have been identified and the mechanism of action is still unclear. It is suggested that sex hormone binding globulin (SHBG), aromatase, epidermal growth factor, and prostate steroid membrane receptors are involved in the anti-prostatic effect, but less likely that 5alpha-reductase or androgen receptors are involved. It has been shown to inhibit cell proliferation. In addition, stinging nettle can reduce the symptoms of BPH shown in several open studies. This botanical can interfere with numerous medications, from blood-thinning drugs to diuretics and blood pressure medications. Therefore, consider all medications before starting this herb. Occasional side effects include diarrhea and other gastrointestinal problems and sweating. Dose: 120 mg three times a day.

BREAST CANCER IN MALES

Yes. Men can get breast cancer. Male breast cancer is a rare disease, accounting for less than 1 percent of all breast cancer diagnoses worldwide. The cause of breast cancer in males is multifactorial. Occupational risks include high temperature environments and exhaust fumes. High estrogen levels resulting from Klinefelter's, gonadal dysfunction, obesity, or excess alcohol intake also increase your risk as does exposure to radiation, whereas gynecomastia (enlarged breast tissue) does not.

Familial cases usually have BRCA2 rather than BRCA1 mutations. A positive family history increases the relative risk 2.5 times, and 20 percent of men with breast cancer have a first degree relative with the same disease. The left breast is involved more frequently than the right; 1 percent of the cases are bilateral (in both breasts). The most common presentations are a painless palpable mass, skin ulceration, nipple retraction or discharge in approximately 75 percent of the cases, which is very similar to what women experience.

Fortunately, the rate of presentation with advanced stage breast cancer has been decreasing in men. As a matter of fact, a study conducted in 1995 reported the rate of Stage 1 to 2 disease on diagnosis as 70 percent, whereas it was reported as 67 percent in 2010 and 82 percent in 2015. Most tumors are ductal and 10 percent are ductal carcinoma in situ (DCIS), which is the earliest form of breast cancer.

Although mammography, ultrasonography, and scintigraphy can be useful tools in diagnosis; clinical assessment, along with a confirmatory biopsy, remains the main step in the evaluation of men with breast lesions.

Surgery is usually mastectomy with axillary (underarm lymph nodes) clearance or sentinel node (first lymph nodes where cancer cells might spread from a tumor) biopsy. Indications for radiotherapy, by stage, are similar to female breast cancer. Because 90 percent of tumors are estrogen-receptor-positive, tamoxifen is standard adjuvant therapy, but some individuals can also benefit from chemotherapy.

National initiatives are increasingly needed to improve information and support for male breast cancer patients. Reconstructions for restoring body image have been recently reported. In one study, the overall estimated long-term survival was about 90 percent at 5 years, 80 percent at 10 years, and 70 percent at 20 years. Patients carrying a BRCA mutation had a significantly lower survival.

DIABETES

More than 80 percent of the population in the U.S. that are adults have blood glucose levels that are too high. Ten million people in the U.S. have diabetes; another one-half million are believed to be undiagnosed. People with hypertension have a two-fold higher prevalence of diabetes and obesity, half are insulin-resistant. Likewise, patients who are obese are twice as likely to have hypertension, hypertriglyceridemia (high triglycerides), or type II diabetes.

■ Disorders Associated With Diabetes

If an individual has diabetes, they have an increased risk in developing the following diseases.

- **Cancer.** Researchers in one study found men with diabetes had a 34 percent increased risk of developing cancer. The higher risks were linked with a range of cancer types. Men had a significantly higher risk—almost double—for prostate cancer. In addition, type 2 diabetes was also linked with higher risks of leukemia, skin cancer, thyroid cancer, lymphoma, kidney cancer, liver cancer, pancreatic cancer, lung cancer, colorectal cancer, and stomach cancer. Interestingly, men with diabetes were found to have a lower risk of esophageal cancer.

- **Cardiovascular disease and stroke.** Having a fasting blood sugar (FBS) high normal (over 85 mg/dL) the risk of a person dying of cardiovascular disease is increased by 40 percent. Furthermore, having a FBS high normal (over 85 mg/dL) increases your risk of vascular death. People with high after-meal glucose (101 mg/dL) compared to 83 mg/dL) had a 27 percent increased risk of death from stroke in a medical study.

- **Cognitive decline.** Diabetes is associated with an increased risk of developing Alzheimer's disease of 50 percent to 100 percent. A study showed glucose (blood sugar) at the high end of normal results in significant brain shrinkage. The shrinkage occurs in the hippocampus and amygdala. A study also showed significant brain shrinkage among participants whose blood sugar levels were high but below 110 mg/dL. In fact, high normal levels of FBS may account for a 6 percent to 10 percent decrease in the volume of the hippocampus and amygdala.

- **Hypertension.** High levels of insulin correlate with low sodium in the urine. This leads to an increase in water retention, which makes it harder for blood to flow through the circulatory system which then leads to an increase in blood pressure. Insulin also elevated blood pressure by affecting the elasticity of arterial walls. Insulin alters the mechanical action of the blood vessel walls by acting on smooth muscle cells, stimulating them and making them larger. As smooth muscle cells grow, they make the arterial walls thicker, stiffer, and less supple. This forces the heart to work harder and exert more pressure to force the blood through the narrowed vessels.

Causes of Diabetes

The following are some of the common causes of diabetes which are related to defective insulin secretion by the pancreatic-B cells or the inability of insulin-sensitive tissues to respond appropriately to insulin.

- Abuse of alcohol
- Eating processed foods
- Elevated DHEA levels
- Excessive caffeine intake
- Excessive dieting
- Genetic susceptibility (inherited a gene)
- GI tract is not healthy which promotes dysbiosis where the gut bacteria are altered
- Hypothyroidism
- Increased stress
- Insomnia
- Lack of exercise
- Nicotine

■ Therapies for Diabetes

Conventional Therapies

Conventional therapies for diabetes are centered around exercise and a healthy eating program. If you are overweight, then weight reduction is very beneficial. If these methods are not successful, then medication may be added, which include one of the following classes of drugs:

- Alpha-glucosidase inhibitors
- Biguanides
- Dopamine agonists
- DPP-4 inhibitors
- Glucagon-like peptides
- Meglitinides

- Sodium glucose transporter (SGLT)2 inhibitors

- Sulfonylureas

- Thiazolidinediones

Precision Medicine Therapies

The following are Precision Medicine therapies for diabetes:

- **Exercise.** Lack of exercise is a risk factor for the development of insulin resistance and diabetes in susceptible individuals. Try and exercise four hours a week. If you have not been exercising and you are over the age of 42, see your healthcare provider for a stress test before you begin an exercise program.

- **Good sleep hygiene.** This is very important. If you do not sleep at least six and one-half hours a night and/or do not get restorative sleep, then insulin levels may rise and lead to diabetes.

- **Healthy Eating Program.** Eat a low glycemic index (GI) diet. The GI ranks carbohydrate-containing foods on a scale from 0 to 100 according to the speed with which they enter the bloodstream and raise glucose levels. Foods high on the list increase blood sugar and cause insulin to be elevated which increases the risk of developing diabetes. The glycemic index is affected by the size of the particles into which the food breaks down into. Therefore, the more processed the food or the longer it is cooked, the higher the glycemic index. Whole versus refined grains have been shown to decrease the incidence of diabetes.

The fat content of a food influences its glycemic index. The fat slows down the absorption and therefore lowers its glycemic index. The right balance of saturated to polyunsaturated to monounsaturated fats is important both for the prevention and treatment of diabetes.

A high fiber (soluble fiber) eating pattern helps to control blood sugar. Low fiber intake has been shown to be a risk factor in several studies for the development of diabetes.

Get enough protein in your diet. The protein content of the food also decreases the absorption of sugars and consequently decreases its glycemic load.

Weight loss has been proven to be very beneficial to prevent and control blood sugar.

Good sleep hygiene is critical. Without at least six and one-half hours a night of sleep and/or you do not get restorative sleep, then insulin levels may rise and lead to diabetes.

Nutritional Supplements

Most nutritional supplements can be used with oral hypoglycemic agents (medications that lower blood sugar) provided you have normal liver and kidney function. Check with your compounding pharmacist or healthcare provider if you are unsure of a possible drug-nutrient interaction before using.

- *Alpha lipoic acid (ALA)* is both fat and water soluble and is a broad-spectrum antioxidant. It also functions as a co-enzyme in carbohydrate metabolism. In addition, it slows the development of diabetic neuropathy and can be an effective therapy for diabetic neuropathy in conjunction with lowering blood sugar and other nutrients. Dose: 300 to 400 mg a day.

- *Biotin,* an important B vitamin, is not just for hair and nails. Biotin deficiency results in impaired use of glucose by the body. Biotin is made in your GI tract. Therefore, the best way to have an optimal level is to have optimal gut function. Supplementation may also be helpful. Dose: 1 to 2 mg daily.

- *Chromium* is needed for carbohydrate and lipid metabolism. Elevated glucose, insulin, cholesterol, and triglycerides as well as decreased HDL can be improved with chromium. Dose: 600 micrograms to 1,200 micrograms a day with normal kidney function.

- *Conjugated Linoleic Acid (CLA)* is the only naturally occurring trans-fat. It can improve FBS. Dose: 1,000 mg a day.

- *L-arginine* helps insulin work better in the body. Hence it improves FBS. If you have a heart valve problem, only take under the direction of your doctor. Dose: 1,000 mg a day with normal kidney function.

- *L-carnitine* is an antioxidant that influences free fatty acids in glucose oxidation. It also improves diabetic neuropathy. Dose: 1,000 to 2,000 mg a day with normal kidney function. Have your doctor measure your TMAO level before taking. If it is elevated, you cannot supplement with L-carnitine.

- *L-carnosine* is a nutrient which is a combination of two amino acids, beta-alanine and histidine. It is also an antioxidant and aids the body in preventing glycation. Carnosine is found in the brain, skeletal muscles, heart, and the lens of the eye. Dose: 1,000 mg a day with normal kidney function.

- *L-taurine* is an amino acid. It requires zinc to help function properly. Taurine has a positive effect on controlling glucose in diabetics. Stress depletes the body of taurine! Dose: 1,000 to 2,000 mg a day with normal renal function.

- *Magnesium* functions as an essential cofactor in glucose oxidation, and it also modulates glucose transport across cell membranes. Magnesium deficiency is associated with diabetes. Dose 400 to 600 mg a day of magnesium glycinate or threonate.

- *Omega-3-fatty acids* have a positive effect on blood sugar. Dose: 2,000 mg a day.

- *Vanadium* improves insulin sensitivity. Dose: 10 to 50 micrograms. Do not use doses higher than 50 micrograms since higher doses may exacerbate a bipolar disorder.

- *Vitamin D,* in low levels, is associated with diabetes. Studies have shown that supplementing with vitamin D improves insulin sensitivity and blood sugar. Have your healthcare provider measure your vitamin D level.

- *Vitamin E* improves glucose tolerance. If your vitamin E level is low, you are more likely to develop type 2 diabetes. Dose: 200 to 400 IU a day.

Botanical Supplements

Most botanical supplements can be used with oral hypoglycemic agents (medications) provided you have normal renal and hepatic function. Check with your compounding pharmacists or healthcare provider if you are unsure of a possible drug-botanical interaction before using.

- *Aloe vera* in a single-blind, placebo-controlled trial of diabetics over 2 weeks showed improved blood sugar control.

- *Berberine* (Berberis vulgaris) has been shown to lower blood sugar. Dose: 200 to 500 mg two to three times a day. It can cause GI upset in some people.

- *Bitter Melon* (Momordica charantia) is a tropical fruit widely used in Asia, Africa, and South America. It is also called bitter gourd. The exact mechanism of action is unknown. It has been shown in a medical study to work as well as some medications.

- *Cinnamon, clove, and bay leaves* have insulin-like or insulin-potentiating action. Possible side effects of all of these include the following: GI upset, stomatitis (inflammation of the mouth and lips), and perioral dermatitis.

- *Fenugreek* (Trigonella foenum graecum) seeds have a hypoglycemic effect due to its high content of soluble fiber which decreases the rate of gastric emptying and delays the absorption of glucose from the small intestine. There may be a cross-reaction if you are allergic to chickpeas. The possible side effects of this herb include diarrhea, flatulence, and dizziness. Furthermore, fenugreek preparations can contain coumarin derivatives, which may affect clotting. Minerals and medications should be taken separately from fenugreek-containing products since the fiber in the fenugreek may change the absorption rate. If you are taking thyroid medication, fenugreek may interfere with this drug. Consequently, have your healthcare provider measure thyroid levels on a regular basis.

- *Ginseng* species contains triterpenoid glycosides that lower blood sugar by regulating hepatic (liver) glucose uptake, glycogen synthesis, and insulin release. Ginseng (Panax quinaquefolius—American ginseng) has been shown to reduce blood sugar levels after eating in both type 2 diabetics and non-diabetics. It has been reported to decrease fasting blood sugar and HgA2C. Dose: Panax ginseng: 100 to 400 mg of extract standardized to 4 percent ginsenosides.

- *Green coffee bean extract* has been shown to lower blood sugar as well as lower after-meal glucose surges.

- *Green tea* contains epigallocatechin gallate (EGCG) which enhances insulin's activity. It has been also shown to be a possible therapeutic agent for the prevention of diabetes mellitus progression.

- *Gymnema sylvestre* is an herb endemic to India. The common name is gurmar which means "sugar-destroying." It has been shown in clinical trials to lower blood sugar.

- *Ivy Gourd* (Coccinia indica) is an herb in the cucumber family. It helps insulin by its effects on several pathways in the body. Two studies have shown that ivy gourd had significant glucose-lowering effects. Dose: dried leaves or extracts at doses equivalent to 15 grams a day with meals. There are no known side effects of Ivy gourd.

- *Nopal* (Optunia streptacantha) is also called prickly pear cactus. It is high in fiber and pectin. Studies have shown its hypoglycemic effect.

- *Olive leaf extract* contains oleuropein which has been shown to lower blood sugar. It slows the digestion of starches into simple sugars and slows the absorption of simple sugars from the intestines. Furthermore, it increases the uptake of glucose into tissue from the blood and lowers fasting insulin levels. Dose: 500 mg once or twice a day.

- *Pycnogenol* (Pinus maritima) is a standardized extract of French maritime pine bark. A study was conducted on type II diabetics that were given 125 mg of Pycnogenol a day versus a placebo. The people in the treatment group had lower HgA1C, lower blood pressure and lower LDL than before the study began.

Hormones

Many hormones influence blood sugar in men.

- *Cortisol* levels that are too low or elevated can have a negative impact on blood sugar.

- *DHEA* has been shown to improve insulin sensitivity and consequently the potential to decrease the risk of a person developing diabetes.

- *Testosterone* levels that are low is a risk factor for insulin resistance and diabetes. In fact, male hypogonadism (low testosterone) can affect up to 50 percent of men diagnosed with type 2 diabetes. As you have seen, data suggests that testosterone therapy may have a positive effect on bones, muscles, erythropoiesis and anemia, libido, mood and cognition, penile erection, cholesterol, fasting blood glucose, glycated hemoglobin, insulin resistance, visceral adiposity, and quality of life.

- *Thyroid hormone*, optimal thyroid function, is key to glucose regulation. Both hyper- and hypothyroidism have been associated with insulin resistance which has been reported to be the major cause of impaired glucose metabolism in type 2 diabetes. Moreover, type 2 diabetes reduces thyroid-stimulating hormone (TSH) levels and impairs the conversion of T4 to T3 in peripheral tissues.

GI health is key to the prevention and treatment of type 2 diabetes. Data are accumulating in animal models and human studies suggesting that obesity and type 2 diabetes are associated with profound dysbiosis, where the body produces too much bad bacteria and/or not enough good bacteria. A study demonstrated significant correlations of specific intestinal bacteria, certain bacterial genes, and respective metabolic pathways with type 2 diabetes. In fact, butyrate-producing bacteria, such as Roseburia intestinalis and Faecalibacterium prausnitzii concentrations, were lower in diabetics.

Other studies suggest changing the gut microbiota as a therapeutic target in the context of obesity and type 2 diabetes using probiotics and prebiotic therapies, such as inulin-type fructans, arabinoxylans, chitin glucans, and polyphenols. In another trial, modulation of the gut microbiota (by an increase in the Akkermansia (spp. Population) was suggested to possibly contribute to the antidiabetic effects of the medication metformin, thereby providing a new mechanism for the therapeutic effect of metformin in patients with type 2 diabetes. Consequently, this study and others have suggested that pharmacological manipulation of the gut microbiota in favor of Akkermansia may be a potential treatment for type 2 diabetes.

As you have seen, there are many treatments both conventional and Precision Medicine therapies that have been useful in helping to regulate blood sugar. Often, a combination of modalities is the most effective.

ERECTILE DYSFUNCTION

Erectile dysfunction (ED) is a multidimensional but common male sexual dysfunction that involves an alteration in any of the components of the erectile response. Erectile dysfunction is defined as the persistent inability to achieve or maintain an erection adequate for satisfactory sexual activity. After premature ejaculation, it is the most common disorder of sexual function in men, affecting nearly 30 million individuals in the United States. There is a higher prevalence of erectile dysfunction in the United States and eastern and southeastern Asian countries than in Europe or South America. Owing to its strong association with metabolic syndrome and cardiovascular disease, cardiac assessment may be warranted in men with symptoms of erectile dysfunction.

■ Signs and Symptoms of Erectile Dysfunction

The symptoms of erectile dysfunction are either psychogenic or organic. Current evidence suggests that more than 80 percent of cases have an organic cause.

❏ Psychogenic signs and symptoms

- Excellent nocturnal erection
- Excellent response to phosphodiesterase type 5 inhibitors (medication) is common
- Intermittent function (variability, situational)

- Loss of sustaining capability
- Sudden onset

❏ Organic signs and symptoms

- Gradual onset
- Often progressive
- Consistently poor response
- Erection better in standing position than lying down

Causes of Erectile Dysfunction

While the vast majority of patients with ED will have organic disease, there are usually psychological consequences to ED. Erectile dysfunction can cause considerable emotional damage to the patient and their partner as well as have a significant impact on their quality of life. There are many causes of erectile dysfunction which can be divided into psychogenic etiologies, such as depression or anxiety, and organic erectile dysfunction.

- **Neurogenic.** Neurogenic erectile dysfunction is caused by a deficit in nerve signaling to the corpora cavernosa (the spongy tissue in your penis.) Such deficits can be secondary to spinal cord injury, multiple sclerosis, Parkinson disease, lumbar disc disease, traumatic brain injury, radical pelvic surgery (radical prostatectomy, radical cystectomy, abdominoperineal resection), diabetes, as well as other disease processes.

- **Vasculogenic.** Vascular disease and endothelial dysfunction lead to erectile dysfunction through reduced blood inflow, arterial insufficiency, or arterial stenosis (narrowing of the large arteries). Vasculogenic erectile dysfunction is by far the most common etiology of organic erectile dysfunction. In fact, erectile dysfunction can be a manifestation of an underlying vascular disorder. The risk of developing vasculogenic erectile dysfunction is increased in men with hypertension on anti-hypertensive medication, and for those not on medication, diabetes, and dyslipidemia (abnormal amount of lipids such as cholesterol and triglycerides). Vasculogenic erectile dysfunction does not develop from high blood pressure itself but is secondary to the arterial wall changes (decreased elasticity) in response to the increase in blood pressure. In addition, atherosclerosis related to diabetes, and/or dyslipidemia–imbalance of lipids–can lead to arterial wall changes and compound the vascular injury.

- *Iatrogenic*. The most common iatrogenic (illness caused by medical examination or treatment) cause of erectile dysfunction is radical pelvic surgery. Generally, the damage that occurs during these procedures is primarily neurogenic in nature (cavernous nerve injury), but accessory pudendal artery–supplies blood to the penis– injury can also contribute. In addition, pelvic fractures can cause erectile dysfunction in a similar manner, due to nerve distraction injury and arterial trauma.

- *Medications.* Medication induced erectile dysfunction is an etiology that is commonly overlooked. (See the list of medications associated with erectile dysfunction below.)

- *Endocrine system*. The erectile response to testosterone is partially mediated through sexual desire, but studies have documented a direct role of testosterone on cavernous smooth muscle cells, involving nitric oxide, RHO-associated protein kinase (ROCK), PDE5 and the adrenergic response. Therefore, low testosterone levels are a risk factor for ED.

- *Other hormones*. Little data have addressed the roles of other hormones in erectile dysfunction. Possible roles have been documented for thyroid hormones, prolactin, growth hormone and insulin-like growth factor 1, dehydroepiandrosterone (DHEA), and oxytocin. Although these hormones play a part in the pathophysiology of erection, their epidemiological impact is likely to be small.

Medications Associated with Erectile Dysfunction

- 5-alpha reductase inhibitors used to treat benign prostatic hyperplasia

- Anti-androgens used to treat prostate cancer

- Beta-blockers and spironolactone used to treat hypertension

- Digoxin used to treat atrial fibrillation

- H2 blockers used to treat ulcers

- Luteinizing hormone-releasing agonists and antagonists used to treat prostate cancer

- Opiates used to treat pain

- Thiazide diuretics

- Tricyclic antidepressants, selective serotonin reuptake inhibitors, benzo-diazepines, antipsychotics, and phenytoin used to treat depression and other psychiatric conditions

■ Conditions Associated with or Contributing to Erectile Dysfunction

- **Alcohol Dependence Syndrome.** A study found that erectile dysfunction was common in people with alcohol dependence syndrome. Alcohol abuse is a risk factor for ED. The Centers for Disease Control and Prevention (CDC) recommends that men consume two or fewer alcoholic drinks per day.

- **Inflammation.** Elevated inflammatory markers, such as IL-8 and C-reactive protein, correlate with the severity of erectile dysfunction. This may be related to an increased risk in these individuals of obesity and type 2 diabetes.

- **Metabolic Syndrome.** Erectile dysfunction has recently become a concern as a factor of metabolic syndrome in men. Metabolic syndrome is a cluster of conditions that occur together, increasing your risk of heart disease, stroke, and type 2 diabetes. These conditions include increased blood pressure, high blood sugar, excess body fat around the waist, and abnormal cholesterol and/or triglyceride levels.

- **Smoking.** Cigarette smoking contributes to ED. This may be because smoking can damage blood vessels and prevent enough blood from reaching the penis for an erection. Smoking also reduces the availability of nitric oxide in the body which is needed to cause involuntary muscle relaxation and increased blood flow that play a role in erections. One study found that more frequent smoking was associated with an increased risk of developing ED, as well as more severe erectile dysfunction. Damage from smoking may not be reversible. However, a medical review concluded that quitting smoking, especially for men under age 50, may help improve this disease. There are many successful smoking cessation programs which range from medications, to nutrients, to behavioral therapies.

- **Stress**. Stress and anxiety are often linked to erectile dysfunction. A study conducted in 2019 revealed that stress was one of the main predictors of erectile dysfunction in addition to anxiety and depression. The study suggested that chronic stress may affect testosterone levels or cause insomnia which may contribute to ED. Stress management (see Part I of this book for suggested therapies) has been shown to be beneficial for erectile dysfunction with or without medication.

■ Therapies for Erectile Dysfunction

Conventional Treatments

- Minimally invasive interventions to relieve the symptoms of erectile dysfunction include lifestyle modifications and oral drugs, such PDE5 inhibitors (initially sildenafil, and later, vardenafil, tadalafil, avanafil, and others available outside of the United States). Mechanistically, these drugs competitively inhibit PDE5, leading to a build-up of cGMP upon nitric oxide release, initiating a cascade of events that lead to smooth muscle relaxation and promotion of an erection.

- Sildenafil has been shown to improve erections, leading to successful intercourse in 63 percent of men with general erectile dysfunction compared with 29 percent of men using a placebo. A study in 2001 showed that 59 percent of patients with type 2 diabetes mellitus were able to have successful intercourse while taking sildenafil compared with only 14 percent of those using a placebo.

- In hypogonadal (when your sex glands produce little or no sex hormones) men who have not responded to treatment with PDE5 inhibitors alone, recent studies have suggested that combination of testosterone supplementation and a PDE5 inhibitor can improve erectogenic outcomes. Possible adverse events of this class of drugs include headache, heartburn, facial flushing, nasal congestion, and visual disturbances along with other symptoms.

- Injected vasodilator agents and vacuum erection devices are the next treatment of choice if PDE 5 inhibitors are not successful.

- Lastly, surgical therapies are reserved for the subset of people who have contraindications to these nonsurgical interventions, those who experience adverse effects from (or are refractory to) medical therapy and individuals who also have penile fibrosis or penile vascular insufficiency.

New Therapies for Erectile Dysfunction

What are the latest treatments for erectile dysfunction?

- One of them is penile shockwave therapy or low-intensity extracorporeal shock wave therapy. Shockwave therapy works by improving blood function and encouraging new blood vessels to grow. It does this by pulsing and passing low-intensity sound waves through the erectile tissue. This therapy is still experimental. Therefore, more trials need to be done to assess whether this treatment is safe and effective.

- Another new therapy is in the field of Regenerative Medicine, its goal in treating erectile dysfunction is to change the course of the disease and in many instances to regenerate failing cells, tissues, or whole organ systems. Depending on the severity of tissue damage or the severity of the clinical presentation, various tools, such as growth factors, gene transfer through autologous stem cells where you use your own stem cells to replace damaged or diseased cells, and tissue engineering could be used to achieve this goal.

Precision Medicine Therapies

Precision Medicine Therapies include all of the above therapies plus hormone replacement therapy and nutritional modalities to improve erectile dysfunction.

- **Diet.** Eating a Mediterranean diet has been shown to reduce the risk of developing ED. In addition, other studies have shown that a higher total intake of fruit, a major source of anthocyanins and flavanones, was associated with a 14 percent reduction in the risk of developing erectile dysfunction.

- **Exercise.** Research indicates that physical activity may protect against and improve erectile dysfunction. Moderate-to-intense aerobic exercise four times per week helped reduce ED in medical studies. Physical activity improves the health of your blood vessels, decreases stress, and elevates testosterone levels, all of which can improve this disease.

- **Psychotherapy.** In some cases, erectile dysfunction results from a combination of physical and psychological issues, including fear of failure, sexual trauma, among others. Likewise, erectile dysfunction can lead to anxiety and depression as well as lower self-esteem which can worsen the ED. Psychotherapy may help address these issues. One recent study revealed that psychological interventions such as cognitive behavioral therapy were very effective when paired with medications. Mental health interventions may also be effective on their own for some people. Another recent trial revealed that one month of mindfulness-focused group therapy was beneficial.

- **Sleep.** A study revealed that men who worked night shifts who reported worse sleep quality were at a higher risk of developing ED. Another trial showed that people with a sleep disorder, including insomnia and sleep apnea, had a greater risk of developing this disease. If you do not have good sleep hygiene, your testosterone levels decrease, your blood sugar climbs, as does your blood pressure. All of these are associated with erectile dysfunction.

- **Testosterone Replacement Therapy.** Testosterone replacement may be beneficial for some patients that have low testosterone levels. Part of the erectile response to testosterone is mediated through sexual desire (the male sex drive depends on testosterone), but mechanistic studies have documented a direct role of testosterone on cavernous smooth muscle cells. A recent systematic review and randomized clinical trials revealed that the effects on libido, ejaculation, and sexual activity were apparent within just 2 to 3 weeks of commencing testosterone replacement therapy. The effects on erectile function may take up to 6 to 12 months to be evident.

- **Weight.** In a recent study meta-analysis ED was more common in men who were obese, overweight, or had significantly higher values of BMI. Reducing adiposity—severe or morbidly overweight—is a crucial approach in individuals with erectile dysfunction.

Nutrients

There are several nutrients that have been demonstrated to be effective for erectile dysfunction.

- *Cayenne pepper* is a great proposed remedy for erectile problems. Cayenne pepper boosts the production of nitric oxide in the body and thus helps in achieving firm erections. Also, cayenne pepper lowers blood pressure and facilitates proper blood supply throughout the body.

- *Dark chocolate* is yet another amazing remedy for erectile dysfunction. Dark chocolate contains a number of flavanols and nutrients that aid proper blood flow and reduce blood pressure. It also increases the production of nitric oxide and thus brings about noticeable positive results in the case of erectile dysfunction.

- *Garlic* contains polysulphides. These polysulphides promote the production of hydrogen sulfide (H2S) in the body. H2S improves heart health, relaxes the blood vessels, and lowers blood pressure. Since cardiovascular diseases and hypertension are the leading risk factors for erectile dysfunction, garlic can work wonders in this condition. Studies conducted over the years have revealed that chewing three to four cloves of garlic every day prevents the occurrence of erectile dysfunction episodes. If you are already dealing with erectile problems, raw garlic cloves may bring about significant improvement in the condition within about three months of regular usage.

- *Olive oil* is one of the best home remedies for erectile dysfunction. Researchers suggest that 9 tablespoons of olive oil a week can reduce the risk of erectile dysfunction by about 40 percent.

- *Panax ginseng* has been shown to help ED by improving penile endothelial L-arginine-nitric oxide activity per several medical studies.

- *Pomegranate juice,* in a pilot study, was effective for erectile dysfunction. Other studies have also shown it to be beneficial. In addition, studies have examined the efficacy of pomegranate extracts to improve maladies that are typical risk factors for the development and progression of ED, including hypertension and the ability to inhibit serum angiotensin converting enzyme.

- *Pycnogenol* (French maritime pine bark) and L-arginine combined have been shown to be beneficial in clinical trials. In one study, the combination was more effective than L-arginine alone. After the third month of treatment, 92.5 percent of the men experienced a normal erection. In another study, using the combination of L-arginine and pycnogenol, improvement was observed on hardness of erection and satisfaction with sexual intercourse. In yet another study which was randomized, blinded and placebo-controlled, the administration of pycnogenol improved erectile function in people with diabetes by 45 percent. Dose: Arginine 1,000 mg to 2,000 mg a day. Pyconogenol 40 mg twice a day to three times a day.

- *Resveratrol* improved diabetes-associated erectile dysfunction in lab animals. Moreover, combination therapies with resveratrol and silde-nafil have a synergistic effect in improving ED. In a human trial, res-veratrol preserved the metabolic pathways involved in erectile function and provided functional protection. Resveratrol can also be used as a supplementary agent in individuals undergoing radiotherapy to pre-serve erectile function.

As you have seen, substantial advances have occurred in the under-standing of the pathophysiology of erectile dysfunction that ultimately have led to the development of successful therapies, both conventional and from a Precision Medicine approach.

HEART DISEASE

Heart disease is not a specific disease, but rather a broad term used to describe several diseases that can affect your heart and, in some cases, your blood vessels. Heart disease is also called cardiovascular disease, and can include coronary artery disease (CHD), arrhythmias, blocked vessels that can lead to heart attacks or stroke, heart infections, and heart defects you are born with.

Many people think that if they watch their cholesterol, they will drastically reduce their risk of developing heart disease. However, cholesterol is only part of the picture—one-half of people who die of heart disease has normal cholesterol levels. There are quite a few other risk factors that have to do with adrenal and thyroid hormones, andropause, genetics, and inflammation that men should pay attention to.

Let's begin a look at heart disease related to high cholesterol and elevated triglyceride levels and then progress onto other risk factors for cardiovascular disease.

■ Advanced Cholesterol Profile

It is important that as a man you have the lipoprotein subgroups of cholesterol measured, not just the basic panel, to evaluate new risk factors, which are crucial for an accurate assessment of cardiovascular risk.

This test is called NMR LipoProfile. This is a more accurate way of measuring LDL (bad cholesterol) since it is a direct measure of LDL. A cholesterol panel gives you a calculated measurement. The test also allows for measurement of the lipoprotein subclasses of HDL and LDL.

The NMR® LipoProfile contains the following tests:

- LDL particle number (LDL-P)

- Small LDL particle number (small LDL-P)

- HDL particle number (HDL-P)

- LDL particle size

- A standard cholesterol test (LDL-C, HDL-C, triglycerides, and total cholesterol)

- LP-IR

These subclasses examine particle size and number. If the particle size of cholesterol is small, it is more of a risk factor for heart disease than if the particle size is large. For example, you can have a high HDL (good cholesterol) level, but if the particle size of HDL is mostly small, then your risk for developing heart disease is still increased.

Primary Risk Factors for Heart Disease

Along with elevated cholesterol, some common risk factors for heart disease are:

- **Age.** The older you are, the higher your risk of developing heart disease.

- **Blood pressure.** High blood pressure (hypertension) increases your chance of developing heart disease.

- **Diabetes.** Diabetics have a greater risk of developing heart disease.

- **Diet.** A diet high in fat, salt, or cholesterol can increase your chances of getting heart disease.

- **Gender.** Men are usually at a higher risk of developing heart disease than women.

- **Genetics.** Having heart disease in your family increases your chances of developing the disease.

- **Hygiene.** Poor oral hygiene can lead to infections, which can worsen your risk of developing heart disease.

- **Lack of exercise.** Not exercising increases your risk of developing heart disease.

- **Obesity.** Excess weight increases your chances of developing the disease.

- **Smoking.** Smoking increases your chances of developing the cardiovascular diseases.

- **Stress.** Unresolved stress can damage arteries and worsen other risk factors.

■ Hypercholesterolemia (High Cholesterol)

Cholesterol is a wax-like fatty substance (lipid) found in the cell membranes of all body tissues. About 75 percent of it is synthesized by the body with the remainder being of dietary origin. High-density lipoproteins (HDL) carry cholesterol from the blood to the liver. Low-density lipoproteins (LDL) carry cholesterol from the liver to the remainder of the body. LDL cholesterol particles have more triglycerides and less protein than HDL cholesterol particles. Because they are less dense, LDL particles are also larger than HDL particles. Very low-density lipoprotein (VLDL) particles have the highest ratio of triglycerides to protein and are the largest of the three types of cholesterol.

Cholesterol is important for many biological functions in the body. However, high cholesterol levels, particularly LDL is associated with an increased risk in developing heart disease. Excess triglycerides are also detrimental to your healthy and increase your risk of heart disease. After you eat, and especially if you consume a high-sugar meal, any excess blood sugar that goes unused turns into triglycerides that are then deposited in fat storage areas throughout the body.

What the Cholesterol Ratio?

Sometimes, heart disease risk is assessed using cholesterol ratios. Your healthcare provider will determine a cholesterol ratio by taking your total cholesterol count and dividing it by your HDL cholesterol count. This cholesterol ratio should ideally fall between 1 and 3.5, which signifies that HDL cholesterol comprises a significant portion of your total cholesterol. If your level is above 3.5 you are at a higher risk of developing heart disease.

■ Causes of High Cholesterol

The following are some of the etiologies of hypercholesterolemia:

- Alcoholism
- Amino acid deficiency
- Biotin deficiency
- Carnitine deficiency
- Deficiency of natural antioxidants (such as vitamin E, selenium, and beta-carotene)
- Essential fatty acid deficiency
- Excess dietary starch
- Excess dietary sugar
- Excess hydrogenated or processed fats (such as lard, shortening, cottonseed oil, palm oil, margarine)
- Fiber deficiency
- Food allergies
- Hormone deficiencies (DHEA, testosterone, pregnenolone)
- Hypothyroidism (low thyroid level)
- Increased tissue damage due to infection, radiation, or oxidative activity (free radical production)
- Liver dysfunction
- Medications: Some of which include Cyclosporine, Cimetidine, Antiepileptic drugs, Tamoxifen, Thiazides, Alpha blockers, Retinoids
- Vitamin C deficiency

■ Therapies to Lower Cholesterol

Conventional Therapies

The following are conventional therapies to lower cholesterol:

- Exercise
- High fiber diet
- Medications:
  - Bile acid binding resins

- Cholesterol absorption inhibitors (Ezetimibe)

- Niacin

- Omega-3-fatty acids

- PCSK9 (injectable) inhibitors: Evolocumab, Alirocumab

- Statin drugs

Precision Medicine Therapies

The following are Precision Medicine therapies to lower cholesterol:

- **Amino acids.** Testing amino acids and balancing them according to lab results will help optimize your cholesterol level. Research shows that getting optimal ratios of essential amino acids may play an important role in lowering LDL cholesterol levels and triglycerides. A study found that supplementing with a combination of essential amino acids and phytosterols promoted lower levels of total cholesterol, LDL cholesterol, and triglycerides. Have your doctor order an amino acid test.

- **Balance hormones.** See a Precision Medicine specialist or pharmacist to order salivary testing to test your sex hormones and have them replaced with natural hormones if you are a candidate for testosterone replacement since low testosterone levels are commonly associated with high cholesterol levels. On the salivary test will also be DHEA and cortisol levels. Elevation of either of these hormones can also raise your cholesterol. In addition, make sure that complete thyroid studies have been done since high cholesterol levels may be a manifestation of hypothyroidism (low thyroid function). See Part III of this book for further discussion of testosterone replacement and lowering heart disease risk.

- **Diet.** Eating a diet that is high in soluble fiber will help lower cholesterol. Decrease your intake of trans fats. Add nuts to your diet, such as almonds, walnuts, pecans, pistachios, hazelnuts, and macadamia nuts. Adding sesame seeds to your diet may be beneficial as well. Also add beans to your meal, such as lentils, chickpeas, pinto beans, and navy beans. If you have a normal TAMO (Trimethylamine N-oxide) level (see section on risk factors for heart disease, page 108), most studies have shown that eating up to 28 eggs a week does not raise your cholesterol.

- **Evaluate for infection.** Have your doctor evaluate you for infection. There are two different methods that bacterial and viral infections can raise your cholesterol. One is by altering lipid metabolism which causes your LDL level to rise. Secondly, recent evidence suggests that LDL has antimicrobial properties and LDL is elevated as the body tries to inactivate the pathogens.

- **Exercise.** Exercise helps to lower cholesterol. In fact, the Harvard Alumni Health Study revealed that total physical activity and vigorous activities showed the strongest reductions in CHD risk. The association between physical activity and a reduced risk of heart disease also extended to men with multiple coronary risk factors. Other studies showed that total physical activity, running, weight training, and walking were each associated with reduced CHD risk. Exercising three to four times a week for 20 minutes not only lowers cholesterol, but it will help lower blood sugar and cause weight loss if you are overweight. If you are over 45 and have not been exercising, then see your healthcare provider before you begin an exercise program.

- **Fatty acids.** Fatty acid testing is also an important examination to have your doctor perform to help lower your cholesterol level. Omega-6-fatty acids, such as safflower oil, soybean oil, and sunflower oil, can help decrease cholesterol as can the all-important omega-3-fatty acids.

- **GI health.** Have your healthcare provider order a gut health test. GI infections, such as H. pylori, parasitic infections, and small intestinal small overgrowth (SIBO), can raise your cholesterol level. Leaky gut is when the gut barrier becomes more permeable to endotoxins such as lipopolysaccharides (LPS). These toxins enter the bloodstream and create an immune response. As part of the body's defense against these toxins, it releases a protein called LPS binding protein which circulates with the LDL, this leads to an up regulation of your LDL levels. Addressing gut bacterial infections and dysbiosis (too much bad bacteria and not enough good bacteria) can decrease cholesterol levels by 30 to 40 points.

- **Nutrients.** Have your healthcare provider order a comprehensive nutritional test to coordinate your nutritional therapy to help lower your cholesterol. The following are nutrients found to be effective in lowering cholesterol:
  - *Artichoke* (Cynara scolymus, Cynara cardunculus) decreases LDL, total cholesterol, and triglycerides. Its components luteolin and chlorogenic acid play a key role.

- *Berberine* induces LDL excretion. It works very effectively. Some individuals may get nausea and loose stools with berberine use. Dose: 200 mg to 500 mg three times a day.

- *Bergamot* (Citrus bergamia) inhibits cholesterol synthesis. It has been shown to be one of the most effective natural ways to lower cholesterol. Dose: 500 mg twice a day.

- *Beta-sitosterol* is a plant sterol. It works by inhibiting intestinal absorption of cholesterol. They are usually taken twice a day.

- *Carnitine* lowers total cholesterol and triglycerides. It also causes a significant reduction of Lp(a) level. In addition, carnitine aids in fat metabolism enhancing the transport of fatty acids into the mitochondria. It likewise raises HDL-C. Ask your doctor to measure your TMAO level before supplementing with carnitine. If your TMAO level is elevated, you cannot take carnitine. Dose: 1,000 to 3,000 mg a day if you have normal kidney function.

- *Chitosan* inhibits cholesterol absorption.

- *Chromium* has been shown to lower total cholesterol and raise HDL-C in some studies. Some trials did not show any benefit of this mineral.

- *Fiber*, the soluble form, as a supplement inhibits cholesterol absorption. Soluble fiber includes pectin, guar gum, mucilage, oats, and psyllium. Dose: 20 to 30 grams a day.

- *Garlic* is one of the best methods to lower your cholesterol since it inhibits cholesterol synthesis. Dose: 10 mg allicin or a total allicin potential of 4,000 micrograms (equal to one clove of garlic) once a day. Garlic is a blood thinner. Do not use if you are taking any kind of blood-thinning medication or supplement.

- *Green tea.* Drinking green tea or taking it as a supplement (EGCG) lowers total cholesterol and LDL-C. Green tea extract can interact with a number of drugs. Check with your healthcare provider before taking this supplement. Dose: 200 to 400 mg twice a day.

- *Gugulipid* lowers cholesterol. Do not take if you are taking a blood thinning medication or a nutrient that causes your blood to thin, since gugulipid has anticoagulant activity. Dose: 50 mg twice a day.

- *Magnesium glycinate* increase HDL-C. It also has many other functions in the body. Dose: 400 to 500 mg a day.

- *Niacin* works by lowering total cholesterol, LDL-C, and triglycerides. It also raises HDL-C. Do not use if you are taking a statin drug. This nutrient in large doses may also raise your blood sugar and can increase your liver enzymes. Dose: 1.5 to 3 grams a day.

- *Pantetheine* inhibits cholesterol synthesis and lowers total cholesterol and triglycerides. It also raises HDL-C. Dose: 900 mg a day.

- *Policosanol* (from sugar cane) inhibits the making of cholesterol by the body. Dose: 10 mg twice a day.

- *Red yeast rice* lowers cholesterol very effectively. It works by inhibiting cholesterol synthesis and improving endothelial (thin membrane inside of heart and blood vessels) function. It lowers both total cholesterol and LDL-C. In addition, it decreases C-reactive protein (CRP). Like statin drugs it can deplete the body of the important nutrient coenzyme Q-10. Therefore, supplement with coenzyme Q-10: 100 mg a day. Do not take red yeast rice with a statin drug. Dose: 600 mg twice a day.

- *Tocotrienols* are natural analogs of vitamin E. Taken twice a day they have been shown to reduce cholesterol levels.

- Targeted probiotics inhibit cholesterol absorption, such as *Lactobacillus reuteri* NCIMB 30242. In addition, keep alcohol intake to a minimum.

Conventional medications may be mixed with Precision Medicine therapies to effectively help you lower cholesterol, except for statin drugs, niacin, and red yeast rice.

Hypertriglyceridemia (High Triglycerides)

Triglycerides are the form that fat takes when it is being stored for energy in the body. High triglyceride levels increase the person's risk of developing heart disease and pancreatitis. Furthermore, elevated triglyceride levels are the second most common dyslipidemic (blood lipid levels that are too high or too low) change in individuals with hypertension after an increase in LDL-C. In addition, hypertriglyceridemia influences the metabolism of other lipoproteins, transport of proteins, enzymes function, coagulation properties, and endothelial dysfunction (damage to the vascular tissue).

Causes of High Triglycerides

High triglycerides tend to show up along with other problems, like high blood pressure, diabetes, obesity, high levels of "bad" LDL cholesterol as you age. It's not uncommon for people with high triglycerides to have more than one cause factoring into their condition. The following can cause or contribute to the rise of triglyceride levels:

- Alcohol
- Caffeine
- Diuretics
- Family inheritance
- Fruit juice
- High fat diet
- Insulin resistance
- Lack of physical activity
- Nephrotic syndrome (kidney disorder)

- Nicotine
- Skipping breakfast and/or lunch and making up for it at supper
- Soft drinks
- Stress
- Too much fruit
- White bread, cakes, cookies, candies
- White flour
- White sugar

■ Ways to Lower Triglyceride Levels

There are many ways to lower high triglyceride levels. Decreasing your intake of fruits to two serving a day and eliminating fruit juices has been shown to be beneficial. Also eating a good fat diet; a low glycemic index (low sugar) eating program has been shown to be helpful. Of course, like many things that can help us be healthier, exercise will lower triglycerides. There are many nutrients that can also lower your triglyceride level. EPA/ DHA (fish oil) has been shown to be the most effective, as well as the nutrients in the table of supplements below.

SUPPLEMENTS THAT DECREASE TRIGLYCERIDES		
Supplements	Dosage	Considerations
Alpha-ketoglutarate	500 to 1,000 mg once a day	Use with caution if you get cold sores.

Arginine	2 to 4 g once a day	If you have kidney disease, liver disease, or herpes, only take under a doctor's supervision.
Chromium	300 mcg once a day	Combining with the protein picolinate allows your body to absorb chromium more efficiently. However, some chromium picolinate supplements contain more chromium than necessary. Ask your healthcare provider for a recommendation on chromium consumption.
Coenzyme Q10	60 to 120 mg once a day	May reduce the effects of blood thinners. May cause diarrhea in dosages above 100 mg once a day.
EPA/DHA (fish oil)	2,000 to 4,000 mg once a day	Choose a source that contains vitamin E to prevent oxidation. Doses of 4,000 mg a day or more act as a blood thinner. Do not take more than 3,000 mg a day if you are taking a prescription blood thinning drug.
Gugulipid	500 to 1,000 mg once a day	
Lysine	1,000 to 3,000 mg once a day	Taking for more than six months can cause an imbalance of arginine. Do not take if you have diabetes or are allergic to eggs, milk, or wheat.
Magnesium	600 mg once a day	Consult healthcare provider for dosage if you have kidney disease. Discontinue use and see your doctor if you experience abdominal pain. Take a lower dose if it causes diarrhea.
Methionine	250 to 500 mg once a day	Take with vitamins B-6 and B-9 to prevent a build-up of homocysteine. May counteract the effects of levodopa (a drug used to treat Parkinson's disease).
Niacin	1 to 2 g once a day	Do not take the suggested dosage without first consulting your doctor. Large dosages can cause a "flush" feeling, which can be eliminated by taking an aspirin one hour before the niacin. Do not drink alcohol or hot drinks within one hour of taking niacin.
Policosanol	10 to 20 mg once a day	
Vitamin B-5 (pantothenic acid)	100 mg once a day	High doses can deplete your body of other vitamins in the B complex.

Vitamin B-9 (folic acid)	1 mg twice a day	High doses can deplete your body of other vitamins in the B complex.
Vitamin E	400 IU once a day	Take tocotrienols, the most active type of vitamin E.
Zinc	25 mg once a day	The best zinc supplements are zinc picolinate and zinc citrate. If you are taking zinc and iron supplements, take one in the morning and one in the evening. (Taking them together reduces the efficiency of both.)

In addition, natural hormone replacement has been shown to lower your triglyceride level.

Since lipids, such as cholesterol and triglycerides, are insoluble in water these lipids must be transported in association with proteins (lipoproteins) in the circulation. Large quantities of fatty acids from meals must be transported as triglycerides to avoid toxicity. These lipoproteins play a key role in the absorption and transport of dietary lipids by the small intestine; in the transport of lipids from the liver to peripheral tissues, and the transport of lipids from peripheral tissues to the liver and intestine (reverse cholesterol transport). A secondary function is to transport toxic foreign hydrophobic (doesn't dissolve easily in water) and amphipathic (contains both water-soluble and not water-soluble) compounds, such as bacterial endotoxin (found in outer membrane of bacteria), from areas of invasion and infection.

To be more specific, cholesterol and triglycerides are insoluble in water and therefore these lipids must be transported in association with proteins. Lipoproteins are complex particles with a central core containing cholesterol esters—chemical compound derived from an acid—and triglycerides surrounded by free cholesterol. These help with the formation and function of substances (lipoprotein) made of protein and fat that carry cholesterol through the bloodstream. Plasma lipoproteins can be divided into seven classes based on size, lipid composition, and if elevated they can increase your risk of heart disease. HDL decreases your risk.

■ Lipoprotein Particles

- *Chylomicrons*. These are large triglyceride rich particles made by the intestine, which are involved in the transport of dietary triglycerides and cholesterol to peripheral tissues and liver. These particles contain apolipoproteins—proteins that bind lipids. The size of chylomicrons varies depending on the amount of fat ingested. A high fat meal leads to the formation of large chylomicron particles due to the increased amount of triglyceride being transported, whereas in the fasting state the chylomicron particles are small carrying decreased quantities of triglyceride.

- *Chylomicron Remnants.* The removal of triglyceride from chylomicrons by peripheral tissues results in smaller particles called chylomicron remnants. Compared to chylomicrons, these particles are enriched in cholesterol and are pro-atherogenic (cause heart disease).

- *Very Low-Density Lipoproteins (VLDL).* These particles are produced by the liver and are triglyceride rich. They contain apolipoprotein. Similar to chylomicrons the size of the VLDL particles can vary depending on the quantity of triglyceride carried in the particle. When triglyceride production in the liver is increased, the secreted VLDL particles are large. However, VLDL particles are smaller than chylomicrons.

- *Intermediate-Density Lipoproteins (IDL; VLDL Remnants).* The removal of triglycerides from VLDL by muscle and adipose tissue—body fat— results in the formation of IDL particles which are enriched in cholesterol. These particles contain apolipoprotein B-100 and E. These IDL particles if elevated increase your risk of heart disease.

- *Low-Density Lipoproteins (LDL).* These particles are derived from VLDL and IDL particles and they are even further enriched in cholesterol. LDL carries the majority of the cholesterol that is in the circulation. LDL consists of a spectrum of particles varying in size and density. An abundance of small dense LDL particles are seen in association with hypertriglyceridemia (high triglycerides), low HDL levels, obesity, type 2 diabetes, infectious and inflammatory states. These small dense LDL particles are considered to be more pro-atherogenic (promoting fatty deposits in the arterial walls) than large LDL particles for a number of reasons. Small dense LDL particles have a decreased affinity for the LDL receptor resulting in a prolonged retention time in the circulation. In addition, they more easily enter the arterial wall and bind more avidly to intra-arterial proteoglycans (compound containing carbohydrate linked to protein), which traps them in the arterial wall. Finally, small dense LDL particles are more susceptible to oxidation, which could result in an enhanced uptake by macrophages—a type of white blood cell.

- *High-Density Lipoproteins (HDL).* These particles play an important role in reverse cholesterol transport from peripheral tissues to the liver, which is one potential mechanism by which HDL may be anti-atherogenic. In addition, HDL particles have antioxidant, anti-inflammatory, anti-thrombotic, and anti-apoptotic (cause cell destruction) properties, which may also contribute to their ability to inhibit atherosclerosis. HDL particles are enriched in cholesterol and phospholipids. Apolipoproteins are associated with these particles. Apo A-I is the core structural protein, and each HDL particle may contain multiple Apo A-I molecules. HDL particles are very heterogeneous and can be classified based on density, size, charge, or apolipoprotein composition.

- *Lipoprotein (a) (Lp (a)).* This particle is pro-atherogenic, and therefore, if elevated increases your risk of developing atherosclerosis. The physiologic function of this lipoprotein is unknown. It is primarily genetically regulated.

- *Apolipoprotein (a).* Apo (a) is synthesized in the liver. High levels of Apo (a) are associated with an increased risk of atherosclerosis. Apo (a) is an inhibitor of fibrinolysis (prevents blood clots from growing) and can also enhance the uptake of lipoproteins by macrophages, both of which could increase the risk of atherosclerosis. The physiologic function of Apo (a) is unknown.

SECONDARY RISK FACTORS FOR HEART DISEASE

It is important that as a man, you also have your secondary risk factors for heart disease measured. The risk factors you need to look out for are elevated levels of homocysteine, iron (ferritin), lipoprotein A, fibrinogen, C-reactive protein, Interleukin 6 (IL-6), and trimethylamine-N-oxide (TMAO).

■ Homocysteine

Homocysteine is an amino acid not supplied by the diet that can be converted into cysteine or recycled into methionine, an essential amino acid, with the aid of specific B vitamins. High levels promote free radical production. Free radicals are molecules that lack an electron. They will search through your body for an electron until they find a healthy cell, and then they steal the healthy cell's electron. This process kills the cell. If enough cells die, it leads to death.

This process is also one of the causes of oxidative stress, which can lead to vascular disease, a condition that affects your circulatory system. Oxidative stress is a term used to describe internal inflammation and the free radicals produced as a result of this inflammation. It is caused by an imbalance between the production of reactive oxygen and the body's ability to detoxify it.

In addition, studies have indicated that elevated homocysteine levels are directly related to strokes, peripheral vascular disease, cardiovascular disease, cognitive decline, osteoporosis, diabetes, and depression. Elevated homocysteine levels have also been associated with several other disease processes, including multiple sclerosis (MS), type-2 diabetes, renal failure, and rheumatoid arthritis. Additionally, elevated homocysteine levels have been associated with an increase in prostate cancer risk as well as erectile dysfunction. When homocysteine levels are greater than normal limits, it signifies a disruption in the metabolism of homocysteine.

Your homocysteine levels may naturally increase with andropause–symptoms men experience as their testosterone levels decrease with age. Therefore, it's good to get your levels checked regularly at that age.

Causes of Excess Homocysteine

- Andropause
- Drugs
- Genetic mutations and enzyme deficiencies
- Hypothyroidism
- Renal failure
- Rich diet
- Smoking
- Toxins

High homocysteine levels can damage the arterial lining of the heart, making it narrow and inelastic (a condition also known as "hardening" of the arteries, or arteriosclerosis). When levels are elevated, homocysteine can reduce nitric oxide production, which can lead to high blood pressure, a risk factor for heart disease. High homocysteine levels also elevate triglyceride and cholesterol synthesis.

Studies suggest that 42 percent of strokes, 28 percent of peripheral vascular disease (which causes leg pain, cramping, and loss of circulation), and approximately 30 percent of cardiovascular disease (heart attacks, chest pain) are directly related to elevated homocysteine levels. Furthermore, a study published in the *New England Journal of Medicine* in July 1997 showed that people with homocysteine levels below nine were much less likely to die. An optimal level of homocysteine is 6 to 8 micromol/L.

In instances where high homocysteine levels are hereditary, it is commonly due to the lack of the enzyme methylenetetrahydrofolate reductase (MTHFR), which breaks down homocysteine. A deficiency of this enzyme increases the need for folate in order to prevent high homocysteine levels. This occurs in 12 percent of the population. Deficiencies of methionine synthase (MS) and cystathionine β-synthase (CβS) also result in elevated homocysteine levels in the body.

Ways to Lower Homocysteine Levels

- Exercise

- Hormone replacement therapy that includes testosterone if you are deficient and a candidate for hormone replacement

- Optimizing thyroid function can lower homocysteine levels

- Improve methylation

- Quit smoking if you smoke cigarettes

- Stress reduction

- Supplementation with vitamins B_6, B_{12}, and folate. As previously stated, your body needs adequate amounts of B_6, B_{12}, and folate to break down homocysteine. B vitamins are water soluble and excessive ingestion of caffeine products, alcohol, or diuretics (water pills) will wash B vitamins out of your system. Some people may still have elevated homocysteine levels after supplementing with B_6, B_{12}, and folate. These people will need to take the active form of folic acid (L-5-MTHF).

  Researchers have suggested that folate supplementation could save 20,000 to 50,000 lives from heart disease every year. In addition to supplementation, folate can be found in dark green leafy vegetables, beans, legumes, and oranges. Some individuals will also need the activated form of B12 (methylcobalamin) and the activated form of B6 (pyridoxal-5-phosphate).

  Consuming broccoli, spinach, and beets also increase the conversion of homocysteine in your body. Likewise, SAM-e (s-adenosylmethionine) will also help break down homocysteine. The suggested dosage is 200 to 400 mg a day.

Garlic at the dosage of 1,000 mg a day and trimethylglycine (TMG) at 500 to 1,000 mg a day have also been found to lower homocysteine levels.

Consult your doctor to consider discontinuing medications that can raise homocysteine levels, such as prescription niacin and some diuretics (water pills).

■ Iron (Ferritin)

Unless your healthcare provider has placed you on an iron supplement, men do not need to take iron. In many cases, if you take iron, your levels will become too high. Studies have shown that too much iron can increase your risk of heart disease. Every 1 percent increase in ferritin (serum iron) causes a 4 percent elevation in risk of heart attack. Thus, continuing iron supplementation if you do not need it may elevate your ferritin level and predispose you to a heart attack. Therefore, it is a good idea to have your ferritin (iron) level measured.

Elevated iron is seen often in individuals with hemochromatosis or hemosiderosis but also in people that have a chronic inflammatory condition. The following are inflammatory conditions associated with iron overload besides heart disease:

- Cancer, such as leukemia, lymphoma, breast
- Hyperthyroidism
- Iron poisoning
- Liver disease

- Metabolic syndrome
- Recent blood transfusion
- Rheumatoid arthritis
- Type 2 diabetes

How to Lower Ferritin Levels

- Donate blood

- Eat egg yolks (Have your healthcare provider measure TMAO levels first. If you have an elevated TMAO level, you should not eat egg yolks.)

- Exercise
- Fiber
- Polyphenolic-containing beverages
  - Black tea
  - Chamomile
  - Cocoa

- Lime flower
- Pennyroyal
- Peppermint tea
- Vervain

- Reduce alcohol intake
- Stop cigarette smoking

In addition, if your iron level is elevated, do not eat foods that are high in iron until your levels are optimized.

Foods Sources of Iron

The following list is reprinted with permission from Jeffrey Bland's *Clinical Nutrition: A Functional Approach*. Foods that contain the most iron are listed first, followed by foods that contain progressively less iron. The listed number describes how many milligrams of iron are in 100 grams (3.5 ounces) of food.

Iron in meat is more bioavailable than iron found in vegetables. Additionally, your body will absorb more iron from vegetables if they are eaten with meat than if they were eaten alone.

100.0 Kelp	3.7 Lean beef	2.1 Lentils
17.3 Brewer's yeast	3.5 Raisins	2.1 Peanuts
16.1 Blackstrap molasses	3.4 Jerusalem artichoke	1.9 Lamb
14.9 Wheat bran	3.4 Brazil nuts	1.9 Tofu
11.2 Pumpkin and squash seeds	3.3 Beet greens	1.8 Green peas
9.4 Wheat germ	3.2 Swiss chard	1.6 Brown rice
8.8 Beef liver	3.1 Dandelion greens	1.6 Ripe olives
7.1 Sunflower seeds	3.1 English walnut	1.5 Chicken
6.8 Millet	3.0 Dates	1.3 Artichoke
6.2 Parsley	2.9 Pork	1.3 Mung bean sprouts
6.1 Clams	2.7 Cooked dry beans	1.2 Salmon
4.7 Almonds	2.4 Sesame seeds, hulled	1.1 Broccoli
3.9 Dried prunes	2.4 Pecans	1.1 Currants
3.8 Cashews	2.3 Eggs	1.1 Whole wheat bread
		1.1 Cauliflower

1.0 Cheddar cheese	0.7 Eggplant	0.5 Brown rice, cooked
1.0 Strawberries	0.7 Sweet potato	0.5 Tomato
1.0 Asparagus	0.6 Avocado	0.4 Orange
0.9 Blackberries	0.6 Figs	0.4 Cherries
0.8 Red cabbage	0.6 Potato	0.4 Summer squash
0.8 Pumpkin	0.6 Corn	0.3 Papaya
0.8 Mushrooms	0.5 Pineapple	0.3 Celery
0.7 Banana	0.5 Nectarine	0.3 Cottage cheese
0.7 Beets	0.5 Watermelon	0.3 Apple
0.7 Carrot	0.5 Winter squash	

■ Lipoprotein (a)

Lipoprotein (a) is a small cholesterol particle that causes inflammation and can clog blood vessels. Research has shown that patients with high lipoprotein (a) have a 70 percent higher risk of developing heart disease over 10 years. High levels of lipoprotein (a) are due to an inherited trait, declining testosterone levels in men at andropause, and statin drug use.

According to the National Lipid Association website lipoprotein (a) is considered elevated at levels greater than 50 mg/DL or 125 nmol/L. There are factors that can affect your test results, such as fever, infection, and recent and considerable weight loss. Therefore, do not have your Lipoprotein (a) level measured if you are running a temperature or are infected.

There are many ways you can lower your lipoprotein (a) level. If you plan to use any of these methods to reduce your levels, be sure to take them daily. You should work with a physician who is familiar with treating high lipoprotein (a) levels to determine which treatment is right for you. Therapies that accelerate LDL clearance and lower LDL levels do not lower Lp (a) levels (for example statin therapy). The kidney appears to play an important role in Lp (a) clearance as kidney disease is associated with delayed clearance and elevations in Lp (a) levels.

Ways to Lower Lipoprotein (a) Levels

- Aged garlic: 1,200 mg twice a day

- Bergamot (Citrus bergamia) inhibits cholesterol synthesis. It has been shown to be one of the most effective natural ways to lower cholesterol. Dose: 500 mg twice a day.

- Coenzyme Q-10: 200 to 300 mg once to twice a day

- Curcumin: 500 mg a day

- EPA/DHA: 1 to 2 grams

- Flax seed

- Ginkgo biloba: 120 mg twice a day

- L-carnitine: 1 to 2 grams in individuals with normal kidney function and normal TMAO levels. L-carnitine should not be taken as a supplement if your TMAO levels are elevated. Therefore, have your healthcare provider measure your TMAO levels before taking this important amino acid.

- L-lysine: 500 to 1,000 mg

- L-proline: 500 to 1,000 mg

- N-acetyl cysteine (NAC): 500 mg to 1,000 mg twice a day. NAC depletes the body of zinc and copper. Therefore, if you are taking NAC long-term, make sure you are also taking a multivitamin. Also take vitamin C 1,000 mg a day to prevent precipitation of cysteine kidney stones if you are supplementing with NAC.

- Niacin: 1 to 2 grams

- Red yeast rice: 600 mg twice a day. Red yeast rice depletes the body of coenzyme Q-10. Therefore, take 100 mg of coenzyme Q-10 once or twice a day in addition to the red yeast rice.

- Resveratrol: 500 mg a day

- Testosterone replacement in men that are candidates for hormone replacement

- Tocotrienols: 400 IU a day

- Vitamin C: 2 to 4 grams

Exercise also effectively lowers high lipoprotein a levels.

For some individuals it is difficult to lower their lipoprotein (a) level.

If that occurs, your doctor may start you on vitamin C, 2,000 mg a day and Nattokinase, 50 mg twice a day. Nattokinase is a blood thinner and therefore you cannot take it if you are on a blood thinner or if you have another reason for increased bleeding.

■ Fibrinogen

Fibrinogen is a clot promoting substance that if elevated is a marker for an increased risk of developing heart disease. Fibrinogen concentrations vary widely among populations and increase with age. People with diabetes, hypertension, and high cholesterol have a higher risk of having elevated fibrinogen levels, as do sedentary and obese individuals.

During andropause, testosterone levels decline. Fibrinogen increases as testosterone decreases so when you are in andropause, your fibrinogen levels can elevate. Research has shown that testosterone replacement therapy can decrease fibrinogen. Additionally, fibrinogen levels also climb if you are a smoker. If you smoke cigarettes, discontinuing smoking is helpful.

Nutritional support includes garlic, cold water fish, vitamin E, ginkgo, and bromelain. In addition, fish oil (EPA/DHA) at 2,000 mg a day has been shown to be effective, as has green tea and ginger. One of the best ways to lower fibrinogen levels is targeted probiotics. A study showed that L. reuteri as a supplement lowered fibrinogen by 14 percent. All of these substances can offset the clotting effects of elevated fibrinogen.

■ C-Reactive Protein

C-reactive protein (hs-CRP) is a marker of inflammation. It is part of the non-specific acute phase response to most forms of inflammation, infection, and tissue damage by activating the complement system and increasing phagocytosis—ingestion of bacteria. It stimulates monocytes to release pro-inflammatory cytokines: IL-1, IL-6, TNF-alpha. Furthermore, CRP stimulates endothelial cells (cells lining the inside of the heart and blood vessels) to express intracellular adhesion molecule (ICAM)-1 and vascular adhesion molecule (VCAM)-1. Decreasing hs-CRP reduces vascular events independent of LDL reduction.

Scientists believe that some infections can cause heart disease. Chlamydia, herpes, and cytomegalovirus, an infection in the herpes group, can cause inflammation in your blood vessels and cause plaque formation, eventually leading to heart disease. Chronic gum disease and an H. pylori infection in your stomach are also causes of inflammation. Elevated levels of C-reactive protein occur when there is inflammation in the body. High levels are a risk factor for heart disease, diabetes, hypertension, depression, peripheral artery disease, congestive heart failure, stroke, atrial fibrillation, and sudden cardiac death.

Since CRP levels can be elevated due to many causes of inflammation, your doctor will want to get a high-sensitivity CRP test (hs-CRP), which is designed for greater accuracy in measuring risk factors for cardiovascular disease. Studies have shown that C-reactive protein can be predictive of future heart attacks, even if you have a normal cholesterol level. Many physicians believe that an elevated CRP level is the most important risk factor for heart disease.

Ways to Lower CRP

- Aged garlic
- Berberine
- Bromelain (do not use of patient is allergic to pineapple)
- Curcumin
- EPA/DHA
- Exercise
- Ginger
- Natural Cox-2 inhibitors: Grapeseed extract (100 to 200 mg/day), Curcumin (300 to 600 mg/day), Green tea (3 cups or 3 capsules/day)
- Quercetin
- Red yeast rice (supplement with Q-10)
- Statin drugs (supplement with Q-10)
- Targeted probiotics. L. reuteri has been shown to lower CRP in a clinical trial. In this study, hs-CRP was decreased by 62 percent.
- Testosterone replacement in men who are candidates for replacement

■ Interleukin-6 (IL-6)

Interleukin-6 (IL-6) is a polypeptide product of monocytes and macrophages. Adipocytes (cells storing fat) also produce IL-6. It is one of more than 30 members of the interleukin family and IL-6 induces the synthesis of C-reactive protein and fibrinogen, which you have seen are risk factors for heart disease.

Causes of Elevated IL-6

The following are causes of elevated IL-6:

- Aging process
- Cigarette smoking
- Excessive alcohol consumption
- Excessive exercising
- Infection
- Insomnia
- Nutrient deficiencies: Vitamin D, zinc, magnesium, calcium, choline
- Poor sleep hygiene
- Stress
- Weight gain

IL-6 stimulates the inflammatory processes in many diseases, for example: diabetes, depression, heart disease, Alzheimer's disease, systemic lupus erythematosus (SLE), multiple myeloma, prostate cancer, rheumatoid arthritis, COVID-19, and Behcet's disease.

Ways to Lower IL-6

- Antidepressants: Imipramine, Venlafaxine

- Botanicals: astragalus, cat's claw, reishi mushroom, red clover, bitter melon, tart cherry, ashwagandha, berberine, hawthorne

- Eating a Mediterranean diet

- Exercise three to four times a week (If you have not been exercising and you are over the age of 40, then see your healthcare provider to have an ECG done before starting an exercise program.)

- Good sleep hygiene

- Medications: Tocilzumab, Metformin, Low dose naltrexone (LDN)

- Optimizing hormone function: leptin, thyroid, melatonin, angiotensin II, cortisol

- Replacing nutritional deficiencies

- Spices: Oregano

- Stop smoking cigarettes

- Supplements: curcumin, EGCG, grape seed extract, phosphatidylcholine, quercetin, MSM, omega-3-fatty acids, schisandra

- Treating infection if present

- Weight loss

■ Trimethylamine-N-Oxide (TMAO)

Studies in diverse populations show that plasma trimethylamine-N-oxide (TMAO) concentrations are positively associated with enhanced atherosclerotic plaques, cardiovascular events, inflammation, type-2 diabetes, central adiposity, hypertension, and inflammatory bowel disease. In addition, TMAO levels that are high are associated with the severity of heart disease along with an increase in mortality. In fact, individuals with high blood levels of TMAO had a four-fold greater risk of dying from any cause over the next five years, one recent study revealed. TMAO is a gut derived metabolite (a substance produced during metabolism). TMAO helps cholesterol attach to the blood vessels. It also makes it harder for the liver and the intestines to get rid of cholesterol. If you have an elevated TMAO blood level, see a Precision Medicine practitioner to order a specialized gut health test to determine if this is the source of your high levels. Individuals with elevated TMAO levels should not eat red meat or egg yolks. They also should not take the supplements choline or carnitine.

As you have seen, there are many risk factors for heart disease. The good news is that most of them can be mitigated using many of the methods described in this section. It may also surprise you to discover that hormones also help prevent and treat caradiovascular disease. See Part III of this book for a discussion of the beneficial effects that hormone replacement has on men in relationship to heart disease.

See **Hypertension.**

HYPERTENSION

According to data from the National Health and Nutrition Examination Survey, overall hypertension prevalence decreased from 47 percent in 1999 to 2000 to 41.7 percent in 2013 to 2014 and then increased to 45.4 percent in 2017 to 2018. In addition, hypertension increased with age: 22.4 percent (aged 18 to 39), 54.5 percent (40 to 59), and 74.5 percent (60 and over).

Systemic arterial hypertension is characterized by persistently high blood pressure in the systemic arteries—branches directly or indirectly from the aorta. Hypertension is commonly expressed as the ratio of the systolic blood pressure (BP) which is the pressure that the blood exerts on the arterial walls when the heart contracts and the diastolic BP which is the pressure when the heart relaxes.

The new American College of Cardiology/American Heart Association guidelines eliminate the classification of prehypertension and divides it into two levels: (1) elevated BP, with a systolic pressure (SBP) between 120 mm Hg and 129 mm Hg and diastolic pressure (DBP) less than 80 mm Hg, and (2) stage 1 hypertension, with an SBP of 130 to 139 mm Hg or a DBP of 80 to 89 mm Hg.

Fewer than half of those with hypertension are aware of their condition, and many others are aware but not treated or inadequately treated. High blood pressure is a major risk factor for coronary heart disease, cerebrovascular disease, kidney disease, and congestive heart failure. In fact, the newest medical literature is discussing what is now called The Hypertension Syndrome which is more than just hypertension. It includes high blood pressure, obesity, decreased arterial compliance, endothelial dysfunction, abnormal glucose metabolism, neurohormonal dysfunction, renal (kidney)-function changes, blood-clotting mechanism changes, abnormal insulin metabolism, left ventricular hypertrophy (enlargement) and dysfunction, accelerated atherogenesis (process of forming plaques in the intima layer of the arteries), and abnormal lipid metabolism.

Causes of Hypertension

There are many contributing factors to hypertension, some of which include the following:

- Diet
- Genetics
- Inflammation
- Lack of exercise
- Lead and/or cadmium exposure
- Low testosterone levels
- Other disease processes, such as:
  - Diabetes
  - Hypercalcemia
  - Hypothyroidism
  - Pheochromocytoma
  - Polyarteritis nodosa
  - Primary hyperaldosteronism

- Renal diseases (kidney diseases)

- Overweight/obesity

- Oxidative stress, which is an imbalance between the production of free radicals and the ability of the body to counteract or detoxify their harmful effects through neutralization by antioxidants.

- Poor sleep hygiene

- Stress

However, most patients with hypertension have essential hypertension where no known cause is present. Individuals with essential hypertension are divided into three categories based on renin activity—measure of the plasma enzyme renin. Renin plays a critical role in vascular reactivity due to its effects in producing the peptide angiotensin II which is vasoconstricting (narrows blood vessels). The secretion of renin is influenced mainly by the person's salt intake and volume status. The categories are:

- Individuals with *low* renin hypertension have low renin activity. Aldosterone—steroid hormone which regulates salt and water in the body—production in these individuals is not being suppressed. This leads to a mild form of hyperaldosteronism (overproduction of aldosterone) resulting in elevated blood pressure. The elevation in blood pressure is due to the retention of sodium being increased along with an increase in fluid volume and blood pressure.

- Individuals with *normal* renin hypertension are commonly insulin resistance and have abdominal obesity. This suggests that there is a relationship between insulin sensitivity and blood pressure. However, hypertension can occur in people that have a normal body weight and do not have non-insulin-dependent diabetes. People with normal renin essential hypertension do not commonly response to sodium restriction.

- *High* renin essential hypertension is less common than other forms of essential hypertension. In this form of high blood pressure high renin levels are associated with hypertension and it is believed to be due to a secondary increase in sympathetic nervous system activation.

If an individual is categorized by renin production, the production of renin may not stay constant.

■ Therapies for Hypertension

Conventional Therapies

Lifestyle Changes

- A healthy eating program is also important. The DASH eating plan encompasses a diet rich in fruits, vegetables, and low-fat dairy products and may lower blood pressure by 8 to 14 mm Hg.

- Exercise is very important to prevent and treat hypertension. Regular aerobic physical activity can facilitate weight loss, decrease BP, and reduce the overall risk of cardiovascular disease. In fact, your blood pressure may be lowered by 4 to 9 mm Hg with moderately intensive physical activity.

- Limiting alcohol intake is also paramount. The consumption of three or more drinks per day is associated with an elevation in blood pressure. Daily alcohol intake should be decreased to less than one ounce of ethanol in man and 0.5 ounces in women. The 2011 ADA standard supports limiting alcohol consumption in patients with diabetes and hypertension.

- Limiting salt intake is key for some people. The American Heart Association recommends that the average daily consumption of sodium chloride not to exceed 6 grams. This may lower blood pressure by 2 to 8 mm Hg.

- Nutrients have also been shown in clinical trials to improve blood pressure. Potassium and magnesium are particularly important. However, you can have side effects if you take too much of either of these nutrients. Have your doctor measure your potassium level which is part of your electrolyte studies. Magnesium is best measured as RBC magnesium which is the amount of magnesium in your red blood cells.

- Weight loss if overweight. Up to 60 percent of all individuals with hypertension are more than 20 percent overweight.

Medications

- Ace inhibitors (ACE)
- Alpha-adrenergic blockers

- Angiotensin receptor blockers (ARBs)
- Beta-adrenergic blockers
  - Beta-adrenergic blockers with alpha-blocking properties
  - Beta-adrenergic blockers with intrinsic sympathomimetic activity
  - Beta-adrenergic blockers with nitric oxide-mediated vasodilating activity
  - Traditional beta-adrenergic blockers
- Calcium channel blockers
  - Dihydropyridines
  - Non-dihydropyridines
- Central alpha-adrenergic agonists
- Combination drugs
- Direct renin inhibitor
- Direct vasodilators
- Diuretics
  - Aldosterone antagonists
  - Loop diuretics
  - Potassium-sparing
  - Thiazide and thiazide-like

The updated Eighth Joint National Committee (JNC 8) guidelines no longer recommend only thiazide-type diuretics as the initial therapy in most patients. According to the JNC 8 guidelines, angiotensin-converting enzyme inhibitors (ACEIs /angiotensin receptor blockers (ARBs), calcium channel blockers (CCBs), and thiazide diuretics are equally effective in hypertensive non-black patients, whereas CCBs and thiazide diuretics are favored in black patients with hypertension. Some new studies suggest that thiazine diuretics should be eliminated as a treatment course.

Precision Medicine Therapies

The following are Precision Medicine therapies for hypertension.

Lifestyle Changes

- A healthy eating program is very important to help regulate your blood pressure. The following are some important ways to change your diet to help with blood pressure control.

  - A raw food diet aids in lowering blood pressure.

  - A small amount of dark chocolate lowers blood pressure. White and milk chocolate do not.

  - Avoid artificial sweeteners.

  - Adding extra virgin olive oil to the diet is also beneficial.

  - Avoid foods you are allergic to. Studies have shown that food allergy contributes to hypertension.

  - Celery has been shown to lower blood pressure since it contains apigenin. Celery is a diuretic (increase the excretion of water from your body), angiotensin II receptor blocker, central alpha agonist, and calcium channel blocker. All of these methods help lower blood pressure. Dose: 4 stalks of celery a day, or 8 tsp. of celery juice three times a day, or 1,000 mg of celery seed extract twice a day, or ½ to 1 tsp. of celery oil three times a day in tincture form.

  - Crude onion extract has been shown to decrease blood pressure.

  - Garlic: raw, powdered, aqueous extract, or other preparations have been shown to lower blood pressure. Garlic is a direct vasodilator, calcium channel blocker, ACE inhibitor, angiotensin II receptor blocker, and central alpha agonist. All of these mechanisms help to lower your blood pressure. Dose: 10,000 micrograms of allicin per day which is equal to four cloves of garlic (4 grams).

  - Increasing dietary fiber has been shown to lower blood pressure.

  - Limiting caffeine intake is beneficial.

  - Limiting sugar intake helps to control blood pressure.

  - Milled flaxseed effectively reduces blood pressure.

  - Pomegranate juice, 2 to 4 ounces a day, is beneficial.

  - The DASH diet has been shown to lower BP.

  - The Mediterranean diet has also been shown to lower BP.

  - Whole oats added to the diet lowers blood pressure.

- Exercise is beneficial to help control blood pressure. One study revealed that approximately 75 percent of people with hypertension were able to lower their blood pressure with a regular exercise program.

- Limiting salt intake is also productive. Avoid high salt foods and try not to add additional salt to your diet.

- Minimize your intake of high fructose corn syrup which is the sweetener in most packaged products. High fructose corn syrup has been shown to increase blood pressure through several mechanisms. It up regulates sodium and chloride receptors that increase intravascular volume, increases sympathetic system nervous system activity, increases vasoconstrictors and blocks vasodilators, decreases nitric oxide, causes endothelial dysfunction, along with other mechanisms which drive up blood pressure.

- Reducing your alcohol consumption will lower your blood pressure if you are drinking excessively.

- Stress reduction lowers blood pressure. Have your healthcare provider measure your cortisol levels and treat according to lab. See section on cortisol, page 24.

- Smoking cessation lowers blood pressure in many patients.

- Weight loss if you are overweight will help lower blood pressure in almost everyone. One study showed that weight loss was as effect as metoprolol (BP medication) in controlling blood pressure.

Nutrients and Herbal Therapies

- *Aged garlic* lowers blood pressure. Dose: 600 mg twice a day.

- *Alpha lipoic acid* has been shown to lower blood pressure since it is a natural calcium channel blocker and direct vasodilator. It also lowers BP through several other mechanisms including reducing oxidative stress and improving mitochondrial function. Dose: 100 to 200 mg a day.

- *B vitamins* such as riboflavin also have a positive effect on blood pressure. Dose: 500 to 750 mg a day. Folic acid is another B vitamin that studies have shown lowers blood pressure. In addition, vitamin B6 is effective to lower BP by acting as a diuretic, calcium channel blocker, angiotensin II receptor blocker, and central alpha agonist. Dose: 50 mg twice a day.

- *Calcium* lowers BP by acting as a diuretic, calcium channel blocker, and direct vasodilator. However, some studies show that taking calcium does not have an influence on blood pressure.

- *Coenzyme Q-10* supplementation lowers blood pressure by acting as a diuretic, angiotensin II receptor blocker, central alpha agonist, and direct vasodilator. Patients with essential hypertension have been shown to have lower Q-10 levels than controls. Dose is 100 to 200 mg a day.

- *Flavonoids,* such as quercetin, have been shown to lower blood pressure by functioning as an angiotensin II blocker and vasodilator. Dose: 150 to 750 mg a day. Hesperidin has also been shown to lower BP. Dose: 250 to 500 mg three times a day.

- *Grape seed extract* has a high phenolic content in the seeds that increases nitric oxide and lowers blood pressure. In studies, grape seed extract has been shown to lower both systolic and diastolic blood pressure. Dose: 500 mg twice a day.

- *Guizhi decoction* (GZD) contains 112 active ingredients. It is a classical Chinese herbal formula to treat hypertension and is now being evaluated in clinical animal trials. The potential mechanisms and therapeutic effects of GZD on hypertension may be attributed to the regulation of cardiac inflammation and fibrosis.

- *Hawthorne berry* lowers blood pressure since it functions as an ace inhibitor, diuretic, and calcium channel blocker. Dose: 160 to 900 mg a day.

- *Hibiscus sabdariffa*. Medical studies have shown that hibiscus tea and Hibiscus extracts have anti-hypertensive affects. Dose: 250 mg of total anthocyanins a day or a tea preparation three times a day.

- *L-arginine* is an amino acid and is a precursor to nitric oxide which is a vasodilator. Dose: 2,000 mg three times a day up to 6,000 mg three times a day. Do not use if you have heart valve abnormalities without seeing your cardiologist.

- *L-carnitine* has been shown to lower BP by acting as a diuretic. Dose:

1,000 mg twice a day. Do not supplement with L-carnitine without seeing your healthcare provider to have your TMAO level measured. If you have an elevated TMAO level, then you are not a candidate to take carnitine.

- *Magnesium* has been shown in medical studies to lower blood pressure by acting as a diuretic, calcium channel blocker, and direct vasodilator. Magnesium glycinate or threonate are the best forms to use. Dose: 400 to 600 mg a day. Not all studies reveal a blood pressure lower effect with the use of magnesium.

- *N-acetyl cysteine* (NAC) lowers blood pressure by decreasing arterial resistance and functioning as a natural calcium channel blocker. Dose: 500 mg twice a day. Long-term use of NAC depletes the body of zinc and copper. Therefore, make sure you also take a multivitamin. If you are prone to cysteine kidney stones, then take 1,000 a day of vitamin C to help prevent stone formation.

- *Olive leaf extract* lowers blood pressure by functioning as an ACE inhibitor. It contains compounds called secoiridoid glycosides. Dose: 1,000 mg a day standardized to 16 percent oleuropein.

- *Omega-3-fatty acids* are one of the best document nutrients that have an anti-hypertensive effect. Many studies have shown that supplementing with fish oil lowers blood pressure by functioning as a direct vasodilator, ACE inhibitor, central alpha agonist, and calcium channel blocker. Omega-3-fatty acids also decrease blood viscosity.

- *Omega-6-fatty* acids, in the form of gamma alpha linoleic acid (GLA), lower blood pressure by promoting the blood vessels to dilate. They also functions as a diuretic, central alpha agonist, and angiotensin II receptor blocker. Safflower oil or sunflower oil are the most common forms of GLA used to control hypertension.

- *Potassium* has been shown to lower both systolic and diastolic blood pressure. It also aids in balancing the hypertensive effects of sodium. Potassium functions as a diuretic, direct vasodilator, central alpha agonist, and angiotensin II receptor blocker. All these mechanisms aid in reducing hypertension. Have your healthcare provider measure your potassium level since you can have side effects if you take too much potassium.

- *Pycnogenol* has been shown in clinical trials to lower blood pressure by reducing serum thromboxane B2 levels. It also protects the cell membranes from oxidative stress, increases ACE inhibitor action, increases vitamin C levels, and increases nitric oxide. Dose: 200 mg a day.

- *Taurine* has been shown to lower blood pressure by functioning as a diuretic, direct vasodilator, and central alpha agonist. Dose: 1,000 to 2,000 mg twice a day.

- *Tomato extract* contains lycopene which is a therapy for hypertension. Dose: 250 mg a day of tomato extract that contains 15 mg of lycopene.

- *Vitamin C* has been shown to decrease blood pressure by lowering oxidative stress and arterial stiffness. It also functions as a diuretic, direct vasodilator, angiotensin II receptor blocker, central alpha agonist, and calcium channel blocker. Dose: 400 to 1,000 mg a day.

- *Vitamin D* has a positive effect on blood pressure according to most clinical trials. Some studies did not show any effect. Have your doctor measure your vitamin D level so that you know the best dose to take.

- *Zinc* has been shown to lower blood pressure by inhibiting the expression of unfavorable genes, improving insulin resistance, and inhibiting the renin-angiotensin-aldosterone system. Dose: 25 mg a day. Zinc and copper need to balance in the body: 10 to 15 mg of zinc to 1 mg of copper.

Hormones

- *Male hormones.* Optimizing and balancing testosterone aids in lowering both diastolic and systolic blood pressure in men.

- *Thyroid hormones* must be functioning optimally in order to control your blood pressure. One of the symptoms of low thyroid function (hypothyroidism) is hypertension. See the section on thyroid hormones beginning on page 59. In fact, one study even showed that patients with subclinical hypothyroidism are at a higher risk of developing high blood pressure and dyslipidemia—high level of lipids— compared to controls. Have your doctor measure all the thyroid studies discussed in the chapter on thyroid hormones.

- *Cortisol.* An optimized cortisol level has been shown to lower blood pressure.

- *Insulin* is the hormone that regulates your blood sugar. Insulin also increases the retention of sodium in the body which increases blood volume and drives up blood pressure. Normalizing blood sugar and insulin levels aids in controlling your blood pressure. See the section on insulin beginning on page 48.

- *Melatonin* is the hormone that helps you sleep. However, it also has been shown to lower night-time blood pressure by dilating blood vessels and inhibiting signals from the sympathetic nervous system. In addition, melatonin has proven to lower the high blood pressure that is caused by poor diet choices. It has been shown to protect the kidneys and other organs from long-term consequences of elevated blood pressure. Likewise, controlled release melatonin has been revealed to lower both systolic and diastolic blood pressure.

Other Therapies

- *Stevioside* is a constituent of Stevia rebaudiana (Stevia). It has-been shown to lower blood pressure since it is a natural calcium channel blocker. Dose: 750 to 1,500 mg a day.

See Heart Disease.

MALE INFERTILITY

Physiologic functioning of the testes is essential for male fertility and male secondary sex characteristic development. In men, the primary purposes of the testicles can be summarized as: 1) the production of testosterone and 2) spermatogenesis which is the origin and development of the sperm cells. These critical functions are coordinated through a complex symphony of hormonal signaling known as the hypothalamic-pituitary-gonadal (HPG) axis. Any dysregulation of this pathway can lead to male hypogonadism, infertility, or a combination of these.

In up to 50 percent of cases, infertility issues stem solely from the male. According to some studies, the quality of human semen has deteriorated by 50 percent to 60 percent over the last 40 years. Moreover, recent trials have demonstrated that there is a decline in sperm parameters worldwide in males. These parameters examine semen quality in terms of sperm concentration, motility, and/or morphology. Sperm morphology refers to the shape and size of the sperm as observed under a microscope. It basically examines the shape and appearance of the sperm head, midsection, and tail. The head shape is most important because it carries the genetic information and affects the sperm's ability to dissolve the outer surface of an egg and fertilize it. The mid-piece contains enzyme and multiple mitochondria which supplies energy to the sperm for the journey through the female cervix, uterus, and uterine tubes. The tail is made up of protein fibers and helps the sperm to swim forward in the female genital tract to meet the egg.

■ Causes of Male Infertility

The following are the most common causes of male infertility and change in sperm health.

Environmental Toxins

There are numerous reasons being proposed for this decline. Multiple studies concerning exposure to environmental toxins suggest a negative impact. These toxins may exert estrogenic and/or anti-androgenic effects, which in turn alter the hypothalamic-pituitary-gonadal axis, induce sperm DNA damage, or cause sperm epigenetic changes. Epigenetics examines how the environment can cause changes that affect the way your genes work. In addition, epigenetic changes are reversible and do not change your DNA sequence, but they can change how the body reads a DNA sequence.

Environmental factors that significantly affect male fertility are:

- Age
- Anabolic steroid use
- Cadmium and lead
- Cytotoxic drugs
- Emotional stress
- Environmental pollution
- Excessive alcohol consumption
- Excessive exposure to high temperatures
- Exposure to pesticides and toxins
- Radiofrequency electromagnetic radiation
- Sedentary lifestyle
- Smoking cigarettes and cannabis
- Tight clothing

Understanding the presence and underlying mechanism of these toxins will hopefully help preserve the integrity of the male reproduction system.

Alcohol Consumption. In a medical trial, fifteen cross-sectional studies were included, with 16,395 men enrolled. The results showed that alcohol intake had a detrimental effect on semen volume and normal morphology. The difference was more marked when comparing occasional versus daily consumers, rather than never versus occasional. The results suggested a moderate consumption did not adversely affect semen parameters. Therefore, avoid heavy alcohol drinking. Moderation is the key to health!

Anabolic Steroid Use. Regarding the potential for testicular dysfunction, the threat that anabolic (synthetic) steroid use poses to future fertility and optimal Sertoli and Leydig cell function (Sertoli cells support the production of testosterone by the Leydig cells) cannot be overstated. Multiple studies have documented long-term hypogonadism stemming from prior anabolic steroid use. One survey revealed that the number one regret amongst prior anabolic steroid users was not understanding the potential ramifications that their anabolic steroid use may have on future fertility. Although testicular failure from prior anabolic steroid use has been shown to be treatable in the majority of cases, success is not guaranteed and men desiring future fertility need to be aware of this risk along with other negative impacts that anabolic steroid use has on the body.

Caffeine. One study examined 28 papers reporting observational information on coffee/caffeine intake and reproductive outcomes. Overall, they included 19,967 men. Semen parameters did not seem to be affected by caffeine intake, at least caffeine from coffee, tea, and cocoa drinks, in most studies. Conversely, other contributions suggested a negative effect of cola-containing beverages and caffeine-containing soft drinks on semen volume, count, and concentration. As to regards to sperm DNA defects, caffeine intake seemed associated with aneuploidy–the presence of an abnormal number of chromosomes in a cell–and DNA breaks, but not with other markers of DNA damage. In other words, the literature suggests that caffeine intake, possibly through sperm DNA damage, may negatively affect male reproductive function. Evidence from epidemiological studies on semen parameters and fertility is however inconsistent and inconclusive. Therefore, until further studies are done, try and keep your caffeine intake to two cups of coffee, tea, or iced tea a day.

Cadmium and Lead. Cadmium is a major environmental toxicant that is released into the atmosphere, water, and soil in the form of cadmium oxide, cadmium chloride, or cadmium sulfide. It is released via industrial activities, such as the manufacturing of batteries and pigments, metal smelting refining, and municipal waste incineration. Cigarette smoking also enhances the levels of cadmium and lead. Studies have shown that exposure to cadmium can have possible hazardous effects on sperm quality. In another study, a negative association between seminal lead or cadmium concentration and sperm concentration, sperm motility, and percent of abnormal spermatozoa was found.

Cytotoxic Drugs. Cytotoxic drugs such as chemotherapy, as well as non-cytotoxic drugs, such as tramadol, opioids, and sulfasalazine along with many other medications may have a negative impact on fertility in males. In fact, one study revealed that there were over 65 labels for drugs of various classes that showed that they have the potential to affect human sperm production and maturation. Therefore, when a reprotoxic treatment cannot be stopped and/or when the impact on semen parameters/sperm DNA is potentially irreversible, the cryopreservation of spermatozoa before treatment should be proposed. A reprotoxic treatment is one in which chemical substances that are harmful to reproduction and may cause adverse non-hereditary affect to one's children.

Diet. A high-fat diet resulting from an unhealthy lifestyle, affects the structure of spermatozoa, and also the development of offspring and their health in later stages of life. In addition, healthy dietary models clearly correlate with better sperm quality and a smaller risk of abnormalities in parameters, such as sperm count, sperm concentration and motility, and lower sperm DNA fragmentation.

Exposure to Pesticides and Toxins. Pesticides and toxins play a major role in sperm health.

Nineteen studies assessing environmental or occupational pesticide exposure and sperm parameters were examined in one study from 14 different countries. Seventy-nine percent of the studies found at least one significant association between pesticide exposure and reduced sperm quality. The studies reviewed showed consistent associations between pesticide exposure and diminished sperm parameters, particularly sperm motility and sperm DNA integrity. The findings were consistent with results of previous reviews. After thirty years of mounting evidence, the authors suggested that actions were needed to reduce pesticide risks to testicular function and male fertility.

In another review, the medical literature was searched for studies published between January 2007 and August 2012 that focused on environmental or occupational pesticide exposures. Included in the review are 17 studies, 15 of which reported significant associations between exposure to pesticides and semen quality indicators. Two studies also investigated the roles genetic polymorphisms (alteration in DNA sequence) may play in the strength or directions of these associations. Specific pesticides targeted for study included dichlorodiphenyltrichloroethane (DDT), hexachlorocyclohexane (HCH), and abamectin. Pyrethroids and organophosphates were analyzed as classes of pesticides. Overall, a majority of the studies reported significant associations between pesticide exposure and sperm parameters which compromise sperm health.

In yet another study, it revealed that the pyrethroid (man-made pesticides) exposure affected normal sperm morphology and that organophosphates (human made chemicals used to poison insects) had a negative association with spermatogenesis affecting ejaculate volume, sperm count, concentration, and motility.

Moreover, in a subsequent trial, environmental pyrethroids exposure was found to possibly affect semen quality and the level of reproductive hormones.

In addition, epigenetic modifications, which are changes in the gene expression that are not caused by changes in the DNA sequences but are due to other factors, affect spermatogenesis. One article provided a comprehensive review of the epigenetic processes in the testes, correlation of epigenetic aberrations with male infertility, impact of environmental factors on the epigenome and male fertility, and significance of epigenetic changes/aberrations in assisted reproduction related to spermatogenesis, poor semen parameters, and male infertility. The literature review suggested a significant impact of epigenetic aberrations (epimutations) on spermatogenesis, and this could lead to male infertility. Epimutations (often hypermethylation) in several genes have been reported in association with poor semen parameters or male infertility. Similarly, endocrine disruptors, such as methoxychlor (an estrogenic pesticide) and vinclozolin (an anti-androgenic fungicide) have been found by experiments on animals to affect epigenetic modifications that may cause spermatogenic defects in subsequent generations.

Furthermore, assisted reproduction procedures that have been considered rather safe, are now being implicated in inducing epigenetic changes that could affect fertility in subsequent generations.

Intestinal Microbiota Disorders and Male Infertility. Researchers investigated the relationship between dysbiosis and infertility in an animal model. Dysbiosis occurs when the gut has too many unhealthy bacteria and not enough good bacteria. This trial suggested that there is a relationship between intestinal dysbiosis and sperm quality and spermatogenesis. Therefore, more studies need to be done to further the existing knowledge on the relationship between intestinal microbiota and infertility.

Obesity. Male obesity is associated with increased incidence of low sperm concentration and low progressively motile sperm count, as shown in numerous trials worldwide. One trial revealed that men presenting with a BMI greater than 25 kg/m (2) have fewer chromatin-intact normal-motile sperm cells per ejaculate. Another study revealed that there was a doubling in abnormally low sperm concentration and total sperm count in overweight or obese men compared with men with normal BMI. Likewise, another trial revealed the percentage of men with abnormal volume, concentration, and total sperm increased with increasing body size. In fact, in obese individuals, disorders of the hypothalamic-pituitary-gonadal axis are observed, as well as elevated estrogen levels with a simultaneous decrease in testosterone, luteinizing hormone (LH), and follicle-stimulating hormone (FSH) levels. These are just a few of the medical trials that found that obesity correlated with abnormal sperm quality. Therefore, to ensure maximum fertility potential, individuals are advised to reduce body weight if they are obese.

Pollution. A number of studies found significant results supporting the evidence that air pollution may affect DNA fragmentation, morphology, and motility. The aim of one study was to conduct a systematic review and meta-analysis to assess current evidence regarding the impact of exposure to tobacco smoke and environmental and occupational pollution on sperm quality in humans. In the meta-analysis, 22 studies were included showing that environmental and occupational pollutants may affect sperm count, volume, concentration, motility, vitality, sperm DNA, and chromatin integrity. All the included articles reported significant alterations in at least one of the outcomes studied in association with at least one of the pollutants studied.

Radiofrequency and Electromagnetic Radiation. An interesting trial showed that certain aspects of cell phone use may negatively affect sperm quality in men by decreasing the semen volume, sperm concentration, or sperm count, thus impairing male fertility.

Sedentary Lifestyle. Occupations that require prolonged sitting (such as driving) can have negative effects on fertility. If you have a sedentary job, make sure take time to have a regular exercise program.

Smoking Cigarettes and Cannabis. A systematic review and meta-analysis comprising 58 to 65 men showed that cigarette smoking is associated with reduced sperm count and motility. Deterioration of semen quality was more pronounced in moderate and heavy smokers. Furthermore, the authors suggested that cigarette smoking has an overall negative effect on semen parameters. In addition, repeated use of drugs, such as cocaine and cannabinoids, are associated with a significant decrease in sperm concentration and urinary testosterone in men.

Stress. A review suggested that higher age, smoking, alcohol consumption, and psychological stress were risk factors for poor semen quality. These results indicated that health programs focusing on lifestyle and psychological health would be helpful for male reproductive health.

Tight Clothing. When it comes to sperm, the problem isn't the constriction that tight garments cause; it's the heat. The testicles function best when they are slightly cooler than body temperature. That's why they hang outside of the body. Tight underwear or pants push the testicles up against the body, subsequently increasing their temperature. This increased temperature causes reductions in sperm count and can also cause a decrease in sperm motility. Several studies have supported this theory that tight garments increase testicular temperatures. Therefore, the testicles should be kept slightly cooler than body temperature for ideal sperm production, and tight underwear and pants should be avoided. The remaining question is whether the temperature increase is enough to make a significant difference. Most studies conducted so far have been small, and more research is still necessary to reach a conclusion. In the meantime, it is suggested not to wear tight clothing.

■ Therapies for Male Infertility

What can be done to improve sperm health? Begin by seeing a fertility specialist. Other forms of treatment from a Precision Medicine/Anti-Aging

Medicine are also available. See Part III of this book for a discussion on HCG and clomiphene. The following section will discuss non-prescription therapies.

Diet. Improving your diet and losing weight, if you are overweight, will improve sperm count, concentration, and motility. Eating a Mediterranean diet has been shown to be beneficial since it is anti-inflammatory. In addition, if your intake more than two drinks a day, decrease your alcohol intake. Also, consume caffeine in moderation only. Drinking caffeine all day long will decrease your semen parameters and fertility. Moderation really is the key to health!

Other Therapies. Limit your exposure to pesticides and toxins. In addition, turn off your cell phone and computer at 7 pm to decrease your exposure to ionizing radiation. Do not use anabolic steroids and wear clothes that are not tight fitting. Moreover, make sure you exercise three to four times a week. If you are taking a cytotoxic drug, speak with your healthcare provider to see if there is another drug you can substitute instead. See a Precision Medicine/Anti-Aging specialist to measure toxic metals in your body. If your cadmium and/or lead levels are elevated, having chelation therapy to remove these toxic substances is sometimes beneficial for fertility. Also, have your doctor or pharmacist order a gut health test to see if your GI tract is healthy. At a minimum start a good pharmaceutical grade probiotic. Furthermore, stress reduction techniques are very important.

Nutrients. Nutrients have likewise been shown to improve fertility and sperm quality since oxidative stress tends to be a primary factor underlying male infertility. Start on a multivitamin. The impact of trace elements and vitamins on male semen are the following:

- *Calcium* is involved in steroidogenesis, sperm hyperactivation, acrosome and sperm quality.

- *Coenzyme Q-10* may also be important in terms of semen quality since it is an antioxidant. This nutrient is also involved in all energy-dependent processes in the body, including sperm motility. One study showed that patients that took Q-10 had better sperm motility compared to a placebo. There are not a lot of foods that contain coenzyme Q-10. Therefore, supplementation is recommended.

- *Copper* is involved in sperm quality.

- *Folic acid* is important in the course of spermatogenesis, particularly when taken with zinc. Eating foods that are high in folic acid is important. Your healthcare provider can measure your folic acid and B12 levels to determine if you are deficient in these important B vitamins and need supplementation.

- *L-carnitine* is an amino acid that has a positive impact on sperm maturation and motility as well as spermatogenesis in terms of providing an energy supply to the sperm. This is achieved by transporting long-chain fatty acids to the mitochondria, which are the energy producing cells of the body. Have your healthcare provide measure your TMAO (trimethylamine N-oxide) level. If it is elevated, this nutrient is not for you.

- *Lycopene* is a powerful antioxidant that belongs to the carotenoid family. It reduces lipoid peroxidation and DNA damage, strengthens the immune system, and increases the number and survival of sperm. A study demonstrated a positive correlation between the consumption of lycopene and normal sperm morphology.

- *Magnesium* is involved in sperm quality and development.

- *Manganese* is also engaged in sperm quality and development.

- *N-acetylcysteine (NAC)* is involved in glutathione synthesis and has the ability to decrease reactive oxygen species that are produced by free radical production. The presence of NAC in the diet of infertile men has been associated with an increased number and motility of spermatozoa and an increased number of normal spermatozoa following three months of supplementation. In addition, a decrease in sperm DNA fragmentation as well as a decrease in FSH and LH, and an increase in testosterone levels have been found.

- *Potassium* is involved in sperm quality and capacitation–which are the physiological changes spermatozoa must undergo in order to have the ability to penetrate and fertilize an egg.

- *Selenium* is part of in sperm development and quality. Selenium is a component of glutathione peroxidase and thus increases the enzymatic antioxidant activity.

- *Sodium* is involved with sperm development, acrosome reaction, sperm capacitation, and sperm quality.

- *Vitamin C* is engaged in antioxidant action and has been shown to help prevent air pollution's negative effect on sperm.

- *Vitamin E* is engrossed in antioxidant action.

- *Zinc* is involved in testicles and sperm development, steroidogenesis, acrosome reaction, chemotaxis, sperm quality, sperm capacitation, and antioxidant action. Therefore, zinc constitutes the basic element in the context of male fertility. It maintains the integrity of the genome in spermatozoa and correct structure. Moreover, according to researchers, zinc is effective in protecting sperm from bacterial and chromosome damage.

As you have seen, there are many factors that affect sperm health and there exist substantial data to suggest a decline in sperm counts over time worldwide. Although causative factors have yet to be fully elucidated, potential causes include; increased rates of obesity, poor diet, and exposure to environmental toxins, tight clothing, air pollution, alcohol abuse as well as other etiologies that have been discussed in this chapter. Fortunately, there are now new therapies including medications and nutrients to improve male fertility.

OSTEOPOROSIS

Osteoporosis is a systemic skeletal disorder characterized by low bone mass and microarchitectural deterioration of bone tissue, with a consequential increase in bone fragility and susceptibility of fracture. It is a disease in which bones become more fragile and more likely to break. If untreated, the disease can progress painlessly until a bone breaks. The most common places patients with osteoporosis experience fractures are the hip, the spine, and the wrists. Mild bone loss is called osteopenia. Major bone loss is called osteoporosis.

Osteoporosis is not just a female disease. One-third of the cases of osteoporosis in the United States are in males. Men have bone loss of about 0.5 percent to 1 percent per year starting at the age of 60. One-half of men who fall and break a hip die within a year. In addition, the rate of hip fracture is projected to increase by 310 percent in men over the next decade.

Bone mineral density is not enough. The strength of bone is also important. Almost fifty percent of bone fractures occur in people who have normal bone density. Bone strength is equally as important as bone density. Bone strength involves geometry, microarchitecture and material properties.

Causes of Osteoporosis

- Abnormal cortisol levels

- Acid-base imbalance is important. A diet higher in fruits and vegetables produces a more alkaline environment which reduces urinary calcium excretion. Furthermore, whether a food is acid or alkaline before it is eaten does not necessarily determine how it contributes to acid-base balance after it is eaten. Moreover, foods that are higher in sulfur amino acids, phosphorus, or chloride (for example meat, grains, nuts, and dairy products) contribute to the acidic load. Likewise, foods that are potassium and magnesium salts of organic acids like fruits and vegetables contribute to the alkali load.

- Andropause. In males, low estradiol levels have been associated with an increased risk of developing osteoporosis. Low testosterone levels are also a major risk factor in the development of this disease.

- Caffeine increases calcium loss. If an individual drinks three cups of coffee daily, they lose 45 mg of calcium. Coffee also contains twenty-nine different acids which also draw calcium out bones. In fact, more than 1,000 over-the-counter medications contain caffeine including weight loss products, cold preparation, pain relievers, and allergy products.

- Calcium deficiency

- Electrolyte balance is also important.

- Excessive alcohol intake

- Excessive intake of vitamin A

- Excessive protein intake

- Excessive zinc supplementation

- Fair complexion

- Fluoride in drinking water

- Genetic predisposition. It is also estimated that 50 percent to 80 percent of the individual variability in bone mass is determined by genetics.

- High fat diets

- Hyperparathyroidism
- Hyperthyroidism
- Lack of exercise
- Medications can also increase the risk of bone loss. The following are some of these medications.
  - Androgen suppressive medications for prostate cancer
  - Aromatase inhibitors
  - Cyclosporine
  - Excessive thyroid medication
  - Gonadotrophin-releasing hormone agonists
  - Isoniazid
  - Lasix
  - Lithium
  - Long term use of PPIs (antacids) was shown in a case-controlled study of over 13,000 people with hip fractures that taking high doses of PPIs for more than a year were 2.6 times more likely to break a hip. Taking modest doses of PPIs regularly for 10 years increased the risk of hip fracture 1.2 to 1.6 times.
  - Medroxyprogesterone
  - Methotrexate
  - SSRIs. The 5-year CAMOS study was conducted on 5,000 adults over the age of 50. The use of SRRIs for at least five years was associated with twice the risk of fractures and a reduction of bone density of 4 percent in the hip and 2.4 percent in the spine.
  - Tetracycline
- Poor diet. The DASH trial revealed that people who ate a diet higher in fruits and vegetables had lower bone turnover markers.
- Soft drink use
- Smoking
- Surgeries. Some surgeries increase the risk of bone loss including total thyroidectomy (complete removal of the thyroid gland) and removal of part, or all, of the intestines including intestinal bypass surgery for weight control.
- Thin bone structure
- Vitamin D deficiency

■ Medical Conditions Commonly Associated With Osteoporosis

- Andropause
- Anorexia nervosa
- Celiac
- COPD
- Crohn's disease
- Cushing's disease
- Diabetes mellitus
- Fat malabsorption
- Gallbladder disease
- History of chronic low back pain for more than ten years
- History of stress fractures

- Hypercalciuria
- Hypochlorhydria
- Kidney disease
- Lactose intolerance
- Multiple myeloma
- Nulliparous (never having given birth)
- Oxidative stress
- Primary biliary cirrhosis
- Rheumatoid arthritis
- Scoliosis

■ Therapies for Osteoporosis

Conventional Therapies

The following are conventional therapies for osteoporosis.

- Bisphosphonates

  Possible Side Effects

  - GI symptoms
  - Increase in hip fracture after five years of use
  - Osteonecrosis of the jawbone (jawbone is exposed)
  - Atrial fibrillation (irregular heartbeat)
  - Hypocalcemia (low calcium level)
  - Acute phase reaction (transient flu-like symptoms)
  - Ocular (eye) side effects
  - Musculoskeletal pain
- Calcium
- Exercise
- Reduce alcohol intake
- Vitamin D

Precision Medicine Therapies

The following are Precision Medicine therapies for osteoporosis.

- Decrease the amount of sugar in your diet. Sugar decreases the rate the body absorbs and increases the elimination of calcium and magnesium which can lead to bone loss.

- Exercise 3 to 4 times a week

- Reduce alcohol intake

- Decrease stress. See the section on cortisol. You can do all of the things suggested in this section, but if you stay stressed you may still break down bone!

- See a Precision Medicine specialist to have your hormones replaced if they are low and you are a candidate for hormone replacement. Studies have found that low testosterone levels in men are associated with an increased risk of hip fracture. Other studies have shown that hormone replacement in men that have low testosterone levels has increased bone density in the spine and hip. In addition, make sure that your healthcare provider also measures your estrone and estradiol levels, since both estrogens are equally as important in helping you maintain bone and decrease your risk of developing osteopenia/osteoporosis.

- 5R program for GI health. If you gut is not healthy it is hard to absorb the minerals and other nutrients, you need to build bone. Likewise, low HCL in the gut decreases absorption of minerals. Have your health care provider order a gut health test to determine the health of your GI tract.

- Nutrients: boron, calcium, copper, magnesium, silicon, strontium, vitamin B6, B12, and folate, vitamin D, vitamin K, zinc

Boron. Boron along with vitamin D increases the mineral content in bone and also increases cartilage formation.

Food Sources of Boron

- Almonds
- Apple
- Broccoli
- Cauliflower
- Dates
- Grapes
- Green leafy vegetables, such as kale
- Hazelnuts
- Honey
- Legumes
- Peaches

- Peanuts
- Pears

- Prunes
- Raisins

- Tomatoes

Copper. Copper should be supplemented if zinc is supplemented.

Calcium. Calcium has many beneficial effects on bone structure. There are several forms.

- Calcium citrate to maintain bone or if the individual has bone loss and has a history of calcium nephrolithiasis (kidney stone).

- Calcium hydroxyapatite if a person has osteopenia or osteoporosis and has no history of calcium related kidney stones.

- Calcium should be taken throughout the day for maximum absorption. The body can only absorb 500 mg at a time.

Factors That Decrease Calcium Absorption

- Andropause
- Aging process
- Caffeine
- Celiac disease
- Chronic alcoholism
- Cigarette smoking (nicotine)
- Glucocorticoid excess
- Hyperthyroidism

- Hypoparathyroidism
- Malabsorptive bariatric surgery
- Oxalate
- Phytate
- Sugar
- Vitamin D deficiency
- Weight loss

Milk is not the best source of calcium since pasteurization destroys up to 32 percent of the available calcium.

Calcium

Calcium is the most abundant mineral in the body. More than 99 percent of the body's calcium is in its bones and teeth. Calcium has many functions in the body, including the important role it plays in supporting bone and tooth structure. Calcium reduces bone loss and decreases bone turnover.

Numerous studies have shown that calcium supplementation can help decrease bone loss by 30 to 50 percent.

Important Facts About Calcium

- Calcium carbonate is not the best form of calcium to use. Calcium citrate or hydroxyapatite are now the preferred forms.

- Calcium intake helps lower cholesterol.

- Calcium is also needed for the absorption of vitamin B12.

- Calcium should be taken throughout the day for maximum absorption because your body can only absorb 500 mg at a time. It is best taken with meals and at bedtime.

- Consuming Tums is not a good way to intake calcium, due to poor absorption.

- Hydrochloric acid, citric acid, glycine, and lysine all help increase calcium absorption.

- Milk is not the best source of calcium since pasteurization destroys up to 32 percent of the available calcium.

- Use only pharmaceutical grade calcium supplements. Lower grade products may be contaminated with lead, mercury, arsenic, aluminum, or cadmium. (For suggestions on companies that use pharmaceutical grade supplements see the Resources section on page–.)

- Vitamin C increases calcium absorption by 100 percent.

- You can take too much calcium

Foods That Decrease Calcium Absorption

- Cocoa, chocolate

- Diet high in breads

- Excessive zinc supplementation

- Heavy exercise

- High fat diet

- High fiber cereals, fiber supplements (wait two hours after eating before taking calcium)

- Rhubarb

- Soft drinks

- Spinach

- Swiss chard

- White flour

- Whole wheat

Factors That Increase Calcium Absorption

- B-cell lymphoma
- Carbohydrates
- Estrogen
- Fat
- Food
- Growth
- Lactation
- Lactose
- Lysine
- Obesity
- Prebiotics
- Pregnancy
- Primary hyperparathyroidism
- Probiotics
- Protein
- Sarcoidosis
- Vitamin C increases calcium absorption by 100 percent.
- Vitamin D

Excessive Calcium Consumption May Have Negative Effects

- Blocks the uptake of manganese in the body
- Can causes kidney stones
- Clog arteries (predisposes to heart disease)
- Decreases iron absorption
- Decreases thyroid function
- Interferes with the absorption of magnesium
- Interferes with the absorption of zinc
- Interferes with the making of vitamin K

Magnesium. Magnesium has 300 functions in the body. It is very much needed for bone health.

- Activates bone-building osteoblasts
- Activates vitamin D
- Aids in parathyroid function (decreases bone break down)
- Helps calcitonin function (increases the absorption of calcium)
- Increases mineralization density
- Increases the absorption of calcium

Food Sources of Magnesium

- Almonds
- Apricots, dried
- Avocados
- Brazil nuts
- Buckwheat
- Cashews
- Cheddar cheese
- Coconut
- Collard leaves
- Corn
- Dandelion greens

- Dark green vegetables
- Dates
- Figs, dried
- Kelp
- Parsley
- Peanuts
- Prunes, dried
- Pumpkin seeds
- Rice, brown
- Rye

- Sesame seeds
- Shrimp
- Soybeans
- Spinach, raw
- Sunflower seeds
- Swiss chard
- Tofu
- Wheat bran
- Wheat germ
- Wheat grain
- Yeast, brewer's

Acid-Creating Foods

The average American diet includes many foods that, once eaten, create acid in your body. If you eat mostly acidic foods and not enough alkaline foods, your body must find alkalizing materials elsewhere to neutralize its pH levels. It often must resort to using the calcium and protein in your bones. As a result, your bones can become weakened, possibly irrevocably, and your body systems can age at an accelerated pace, resulting in a slew of related problems. The following foods create particularly high acidity levels in your body.

- Chocolate
- Dairy products, such as butter, cheese, ice cream, milk, and yogurt
- Drinks, such as beer, black tea, coffee, and soft drinks
- Fish, such as haddock
- Fruit, such as blueberries, cranberries, and dried fruit
- Grains, such as barley, oats, rice, wheat, and white bread
- Honey
- Meat products, such as beef, chicken, ham, turkey, and veal

- Nuts, such as peanuts and walnuts
- Processed soybeans
- Sugar
- Vegetables, such as corn
- White vinegar

Manganese. Manganese is needed for the repair of bones and connective tissue. Excessive calcium supplementation can decrease the absorption of manganese.

Strontium. Strontium is a wonderful trace mineral that promotes bone formation and decreases bone resorption. Studies found a reduction in vertebral fractures of 37 percent and 40 percent and a reduction in non-vertebral fractures of 14 percent and 16 percent. The dose is 2 grams for two years and then discontinue taking it.

Vitamins B6, B12, and folic acid. Vitamins B6, B12, and folic acid are commonly low in individuals with osteoporosis. Low levels of these nutrients are associated with elevated homocysteine levels. High homocysteine interferes with collage cross-linking which leads to a defective bone matrix. Therefore, people with elevated homocysteine levels have an increased risk of developing osteoporosis. For information on homocysteine, see the chapter on secondary risk factors for heart disease.

Vitamin D. Vitamin D is a prohormone with many relationshipss in the body to bone structure.

- 1,25(OH)2D3 has been shown to directly accelerate osteoblast-mediated mineralization by stimulating the production of ALP-positive mature matrix vesicles.

- 1,25(OH)2D3 also has a direct effect on bone resorption since it acts as a calcium-regulating hormone and induces receptor activator of nuclear factor kappa-beta ligand (RANKL) expression in osteoblasts.

- A study concluded that vitamin D supplementation decreased the risk of vertebral fractures by 37 percent and non-vertebral fractures by 23 percent.

- Vitamin D supplementation reduced the relative risk of hip fracture by

26 percent and any non-vertebral fracture by 23 percent compared to taking calcium alone or placebo in another medical trial.

- A study showed a link between deficient levels of vitamin D and premature aging of bone.

- Optimal vitamin D status in most people: 55 to 80 ng/mL (120–160 nmol/L).

- Also have a calcium level ordered by your healthcare provider. If calcium levels are elevated, with your doctor find the cause of the high level. Vitamin D excess alone is rarely the case.

- 25-OH vitamin D levels may be normal in patients who are vitamin D toxic and have high calcium levels due to vitamin D hypersensitivity syndrome. Hypersensitivity syndrome is commonly seen in the following cases: cancer, Crohn's disease, granulomatous diseases, hyperparathyroidism, sarcoid, and tuberculosis.

- Supplementation should be with D3 not D2.

Vitamin K. Vitamin K has six major purposes in the body and there are three forms of vitamin K that the body can take in from the diet. Twenty-five percent of your vitamin K comes from what you eat. Seventy-five percent of vitamin K used by the body is produced in our intestinal tract by friendly bacteria.

- K1: found in plants and some of it converts to K2 in the body.

- K2: (MK-4): found in meats, eggs, and dairy products.

- K3: (MK-7): found in fermented soybeans and other fermented foods.

- Vitamin K is important for bone mineralization. Osteocalcin, the chief bone matrix protein, is a Gla-protein that is dependent on vitamin K to be produced. Low levels of vitamin K impair activation of osteocalcin and decrease the activity of bone-forming cells. Therefore, low intake of vitamin K has been associated with bone loss. The good news is that vitamin K supplementation has been effective in preventing and treating osteoporosis.

- A recent study has shown that daily vitamin K intake must be at least 100 micrograms to maintain optimal bone health.

- The following are causes of vitamin K deficiency.
  - Consumption of medications that cause malabsorption of fat
  - Hydrogenated fat intake
  - Lack of adequate beneficial bacteria in the intestine
  - Lack of dietary intake
  - Use of broad-spectrum antibiotics
- Low bone density has been found in people treated with warfarin. There is an association between fracture risk and warfarin use. Studies have shown a benefit and the safety of patients taking warfarin and low-dose vitamin K (100 micrograms a day). Higher doses of vitamin K cannot be used if you are on a blood thinning medication such as warfarin.
- Vitamin K2-MK7 (also known as vitamin K2-7, the MK7 comes from menaquinone 7) is widely regarded as being the most efficient and effective form of vitamin K2. MK-7 is better absorbed and stays in the body longer. The half-life is 3 days compared to a few hours for other forms of vitamin K. Therefore, consider supplementing with vitamin K2-MK7.

Zinc. Zinc is used in many enzymatic reactions in the body. In fact, 100 enzymes use zinc as a cofactor. It is needed for the formation of bone and skin.

PROSTATE CANCER

Worldwide, prostate cancer is the most commonly diagnosed male malignancy and the fourth leading cause of cancer death in men. In 2018, this amounted to 1,280,000 newly diagnosed cases and 359,000 deaths worldwide. Fortunately, the majority of prostate cancers tend to grow slowly (particularly in older men) and are low-grade with relatively low risk and limited aggressiveness. The overall 5-year survival rate for patients with prostate cancer in the United States is 99 percent. In 2015, there were an estimated 3 million prostate cancer survivors in the United States. This is expected to increase to 4 million by 2025.

Risk Factors for Prostate Cancer

Prostate cancer risk factors include:

- Agent Orange exposure
- Ethnicity
- Hypertension
- Increased height
- Lack of exercise
- Male gender
- Obesity
- Older age
- Persistently elevated testosterone levels
- Positive family history

In the United States, prostate cancer is more common in Black men by more than double the rate than in the general population. Moreover, this disease is less common in men of Asian and Hispanic descent than in Whites. The overall incidence increases as people get older; but fortunately, cancer aggressiveness decreases with age. Ninety-nine percent of all prostate cancers occur in those over the age of 50, but when it occurs in younger men, it can be very aggressive. 5-alpha-reductase inhibitors, such as finasteride and dutasteride, may decrease low-grade cancer incidence, but they do not appear to affect high-grade risk and thus, do not significantly improve survival. These medications will reduce PSA levels by about 50 percent which must be accounted for when comparing sequential PSA readings.

The exact cause of prostate cancer is unknown, but genetics is certainly involved. Genetic background and family history are all known to contribute to prostate cancer risk. Men with a first degree relative (father or brother) with prostate cancer have twice the risk of the general population. In addition, the risk increases with an affected brother more than an affected father.

Patients with a strong family history of prostate cancer tend to present with cancer at a younger age (29 years) and with more locally advanced disease. Men with two, first-degree relatives affected have a five-fold greater risk. They also have a higher risk of biochemical recurrence after radical prostatectomy surgery.

In the United States, prostate cancer is not only more common in Blacks, as mentioned previously, it is more deadly in black men. Moreover, the incidence and mortality for Hispanic men are one third lower than for non-Hispanic whites.

No single gene is responsible for prostate cancer, although many genes have now been implicated. In addition, mutations in BRCA1 and BRCA2 have been associated with prostate cancer as well as breast cancer. P53 mutations in primary prostate cancer are relatively rare and are more frequently seen in metastatic disease. Therefore, p53 mutations are generally considered a late and ominous finding in prostate cancer. In fact, over 100 Single nucleotide polymorphisms (SNPs) and other genes have been linked to an increased risk of prostate cancer. A genetic risk score (GRS), including high risk genetic markers and SNPs, has been proposed to help with risk stratification of prostate cancer especially in families; but this type of testing is not yet ready for individual patient diagnostics in most areas.

■ Prostate Cancer Risks

There are many factors that have been shown to increase your risk of developing prostate cancer.

Agent Orange. Agent Orange (an herbicide) exposure may increase the risk of prostate cancer recurrence, particularly following surgery.

Cigarette smoking. Cigarette smoking increases the risk of the development of prostate cancer.

Diet. Diet plays a major role in whether an individual develops prostate cancer. Increased sugar consumption is associated with an increase in developing prostate and breast cancer. Likewise, prostate cancer is generally linked to the consumption of the typical Western diet. A study suggested that diets high in saturated fat and milk products seem to increase the risk. Whole milk consumption after a diagnosis of prostate cancer has been linked to an increased risk of recurrence, especially in overweight men. Concerning red meat and processed meats, the studies are mixed. Some suggest they have little effect and others suggest increased meat consumption is associated with a higher risk. Fish consumption may lower prostate cancer deaths but does not affect the occurrence rate. Some evidence supports the belief that a vegetarian diet, primarily plant based, lowers the rate of prostate cancer, but this statement is not considered conclusive.

Exercise. Exercise and physical activity are vital components in prostate health for preventing and fighting prostate cancer. Studies have shown that for men with prostate cancer, exercise and an active lifestyle provides a better survival rate than those who do not.

Infections. Infections may be associated with the incidence and development of prostate cancer. Particularly infections with chlamydia, gonorrhea, or syphilis increase the risk of developing this disease. Human Papilloma Virus (HPV) has also been proposed to have a role in prostate cancer incidence, but the evidence for this is inconclusive. In addition, a link between prostate cancer and inflammation has been discovered.

Medications. Prostate cancer is linked to some medications, medical procedures, and medical conditions. Use of statins and metformin may decrease prostate cancer risk as well as NSAIDs, especially those with anti-COX 2 activity. Regular aspirin, now used by an estimated 23.7 million men, also appears to reduce prostate cancer risk. Speak with your healthcare provider to determine if you should take aspirin before starting this over-the-counter medication.

Obesity. Obesity has a positive relationship with prostate cancer since it promotes more aggressive and severe carcinomas. This could be due to changes in the amounts of metabolic and sex steroid hormones, such as estrogen, which enhance prostate cancer risk.

Sexual activity. Multiple lifetime sexual partners or starting sexual activity early increases the risk of prostate cancer. Frequent ejaculation may decrease prostate cancer risk, but reduced ejaculatory frequency is not associated with an increased risk of advanced prostate cancer.

Vasectomy. There was once thought to be an association between vasectomy and prostate cancer; but larger, follow-up studies have failed to confirm any such relationship.

Vitamins. Vitamin supplements do not lower the risk, and in fact, some vitamins may increase it. For example, high calcium intake is associated with advanced prostate cancer. There has also been concern that vitamin E, zinc, and selenium may increase the risk in certain populations. Consequently, it is important to have your levels of these and other nutrients measured by your healthcare provider.

■ Testing Methods to Diagnose Prostate Cancer

- **Elevated Prostate Specific Antigen (PSA) levels** (usually greater than

4 ng/ml) in the blood is how 80 percent of prostate cancers initially present, even though elevated PSA levels alone correctly identify prostate cancer only about 25 percent to 30 percent of the time. The literature recommends at least 2 abnormal PSA levels or the presence of a palpable nodule on a digital rectal exam to justify a biopsy and further investigation. The value of PSA screenings remains controversial due to concerns about possible overtreatment of low-risk cancers, over-diagnosis, complications from "unnecessary biopsies," the presumed "limited" actual survival benefit from early diagnosis and treatment, and the true value of definitive therapy intended to cure. In an attempt to improve on PSA testing alone, many alternative pre-biopsy screening tests are now available.

- **PSA Density** is the total PSA divided by the prostatic volume as determined by MRI or ultrasound. The PSA density is intended to minimize the effect of benign prostatic enlargement. In general, if the PSA density is greater than 0.15, it is considered suggestive of malignancy.

- **PSA Velocity** compares serial, annual PSA serum levels. An annual PSA increase of greater than 0.75 ng/ml or greater than 25 percent suggests a potential cancer of the prostate (total PSA 4 to 10 ng/ml). If the total PSA is 2.6 to 4 ng/ml, then an annual increase of 0.35 ng/ml would be considered suspicious.

- **Prostate Cancer Antigen 3 (PCA3)** is an RNA based genetic test performed from a urine sample obtained immediately after a prostatic massage. PCA3 is a long, non-coding RNA molecule that is overexpressed exclusively in prostatic malignancies. It is upregulated 66- fold in prostate cancers. If PCA3 is elevated, it suggests the presence of prostate cancer. It is more reliable than PSA as it is independent of prostate volume. PCA3 is best used to determine the need for a repeat biopsy after initial negative histology. Serial PCA3 testing may also be helpful in monitoring patients with low-grade prostate cancers on active surveillance.

- **The Prostate Health Index (PHI)** is a blood test that includes free PSA, total PSA, and the [-2] proPSA isoform of free PSA. A formula is used to combine these test results mathematically to give the PHI score. This PHI score appears to be superior to PSA, free and total PSA, and PCA3 in predicting the presence of prostate cancer.

- **Mi-Prostate Score** is a predictive algorithm developed at the University of Michigan. It includes PSA, PCA3 and urine TMPRSS2:ERG (a genetic fusion found in about 50 percent of all prostate cancers). While better than PSA alone, it is currently uncertain if this algorithm significantly outperforms PCA3 alone.

- **The "4K" test** measures serum total PSA, free PSA, intact PSA, and human kallikrein antigen 2. It includes clinical digital rectal exam results as well as information from any prior biopsies. Clinically significant prostate cancer is usually defined as Gleason 3 + 4 = 7 or higher disease. A risk analysis of 10 percent or more would typically suggest proceeding with a biopsy. Interestingly, the "4K" test has not been shown to be any better than PSA testing alone when used for tracking active surveillance patients.

- **"ExoDx Prostate Intelliscore (EPI)"** uses PCA3 and urinary TMPRSS2:ERG to detect clinically significant prostate cancer. The test analyzes exosomal RNA for three biomarkers known to be expressed in the urine of men with high-grade prostate cancer. A proprietary algorithm is then used to assign a risk score that predicts the presence of high-grade (Gleason Score = 7 or higher; or any Gleason Grade = 4 or 5) prostate cancer. Unlike other urine-based tests for prostate cancer, no digital rectal examination or prostatic massage is required. Negative predictive value is 91.3 percent with a sensitivity rating of 91.9 percent.

- **Prostate Urine-based test** measures the urinary mRNA levels of the HOXC6 and DLX1 biomarkers following a prostatic digital rectal exam. Measurements are done utilizing reverse transcriptase quantitative polymerase chain reaction technology. Other clinical information such as age, PSA density, family history, prior biopsy results, and digital rectal examination findings are included in the risk stratification. Results are reported as either:

    Low risk: Very low risk of Gleason 7 or higher disease, where a biopsy may safely be reasonably avoided. Negative predictive value is 99.6 percent for Gleason 8 or higher disease and 98 percent for Gleason 7 or higher.

    Increased risk: A biopsy should be considered due to the increased likelihood of finding clinically significant disease.

- **Prostate Imaging.** Ultrasound and MRI are the main imaging modalities used for initial prostate cancer detection and diagnosis. Prostatic

MRI is becoming a standard imaging modality for the diagnosis of prostate cancer. It can identify and grade suspicious prostate nodules to help with staging and localization, check for extracapsular extension, evaluate the seminal vesicles for possible tumor involvement, and determine enlargement of regional lymph nodes that might indicate early metastatic disease.

Various MRI tissue characteristics ultimately determine the relative cancer risk which is documented in the final report as a PI-RADS (Prostate Imaging-Reporting and Data System) score which is a rating scale for the likelihood that clinically significant prostate cancer is present. It is a 5-number system.

PI-RADS 1	**Very low risk.** Clinically significant cancer is highly unlikely to be present.
PI-RADS 2	**Low risk.** Clinically significant cancer is unlikely to be present.
PI-RADS 3	**Intermediate risk.** Clinically significant cancer may or may not be present.
PI-RADS 4	**High risk.** Clinically significant cancer is likely to be present.
PI-RADS 5	**Very high risk.** Clinically significant cancer is highly likely to be present.

Even in experienced centers of excellence for MRI, the negative predictive value has been reported as low as 72 percent to 76 percent meaning that a negative MRI report will miss about one in four high grade prostate cancers.

For this reason, it has been suggested that a bioassay marker be used for additional confirmatory testing in patients with elevated PSA levels who are not proceeding to a prostatic biopsy based on negative MRI findings. Similarly, before starting individuals with low-risk disease on long term active surveillance, a confirmatory genomic test can be useful to help identify those individuals who are at higher risk prior to any clinical disease progression.

Prostate specific membrane antigen (PSMA) based positron emission tomography (PET) correlated with computed tomography (CT) is rapidly emerging as the gold standard imaging modality for staging of intermediate and advanced prostate cancer. Compared to alternative imaging technologies (CT scan, MRI, Bone Scan), it offers superior sensitivity and specificity for both metastatic lymph node detection and bone metastasis.

- **Biopsy.** If cancer is suspected, a prostate biopsy is usually performed. This is almost always done with transrectal ultrasound guidance to make sure that all areas of the prostate are adequately sampled.

  The most commonly used pattern is to take two specimens from each of three areas (base, mid-gland, and apex) on both sides. This is called a 12-core sextant biopsy. The purpose is to better identify the extent and exact location of the tumor. The only test that can dependably and conclusively confirm a cancer diagnosis is still a biopsy. This remains the recommended standard of care.

- **Differential Diagnosis.** Your healthcare provider will also consider other diagnoses when evaluating your prostate, such as acute bacterial prostatitis, prostatic abscess, chronic bacterial prostatitis, benign prostatic hyperplasia, nonbacterial prostatitis, and tuberculosis of the genitourinary system.

■ Therapies for Prostate Cancer

Conventional Treatment

When the cancer is limited to the prostate, it is considered localized and potentially curable. Multiple management options now exist for men diagnosed with prostate cancer.

- Active surveillance (the serial monitoring for disease progression with the intent to cure) appears to be safe and has become the preferred approach for men with less-aggressive prostate cancer, particularly those with a prostate-specific antigen level of less than 10 ng/mL and Gleason score 3 + 3 tumors.

- Surgery and radiation continue to be curative treatments for localized disease but have adverse effects, such as urinary symptoms and sexual dysfunction, that can negatively affect quality of life.

- If the disease has spread to the bones or elsewhere outside the prostate; pain medications, bisphosphonates, rank ligand inhibitors, hormone treatment, chemotherapy, radiopharmaceuticals, immunotherapy, focused radiation, and other targeted therapies can be used. Outcomes depend on a person's age, associated health problems, tumor histology, and the extent of cancer.

Precision Medicine Therapies

Diet. Diet plays a major role in both the prevention and treatment of prostate cancer. Therefore, consider dietary intervention. A study found significant protective associations for fish and tomato sauce but not raw tomatoes. This may be due to the fact that when the tomatoes are cooked the lycopene is absorbed more readily than when they are raw.

Omega-3 fatty acid intake may be protective, as well as vegetable consumption overall. In contrast, milk was found to increase risk for progressive disease. This supports earlier findings that high calcium intakes, either through dairy products or supplements, may be associated with more aggressive disease.

Interestingly coffee plays a protective role against prostate cancer. The amount is generally considered to be 1 to 2 cups of coffee a day. Moderation is the key to health. Moreover, alcoholic beverages tend to be a significant risk factor for the development of a variety of cancers, including prostate cancer. If you are consuming more than two drinks a day, consider reducing your alcohol intake to decrease your risk of prostate cancer. If you have prostate cancer, then consider not drinking any alcohol since alcohol is high in sugar content. In addition, a study found an increased consumption of sugars from sugar-sweetened beverages was associated with increased risk of prostate cancer for men in the highest quartile of sugar consumption. Consequently, limiting your intake of sugars from beverages may be important in the prevention of prostate cancer. Likewise, the total dietary intake of sugars is independently and positively associated with higher serum PSA concentrations in adult American males who are without a personal history of malignant tumors according to a medical trial. Likewise, a study found that higher intake of fruit juice was associated with a 58 percent increased risk in developing prostate cancer. How much sugar is in a glass of orange juice for example? An 8-ounce glass of 100 percent orange juice contains around 21 grams of natural sugar.

Estrogen. As you have seen in Part I of this text, men make estrogen. High levels of estrogen in men have been identified as a carcinogenic component to prostate cancer. Have your healthcare provider or pharmacist measure your estradiol level and estrone levels to determine if your body is making the right amount of estrogens and work with them to help lower your levels if they are elevated.

Exercise. Physical activity may compensate for the effects of obesity by reversing some of the detrimental mechanisms that lead to prostate cancer development.

Smoking Cessation. If you smoke, work with your healthcare provider to try and stop smoking. There are many excellent smoking cessation programs now available.

Low-Dose Naltrexone (LDN). When substantial numbers of leukocytes were discovered in carcinoma biopsies, a link between prostate cancer and inflammation was discovered. In clinical trials, lifestyle modifications, including healthy diet, exercise, alcohol, and smoking cessation, have proven effective in ameliorating inflammation and reducing the risk of cancer-related deaths. Low-dose naltrexone operates as a novel anti-inflammatory agent in the central nervous system, via action on microglial cells. These effects are unique to low dosages of naltrexone and appear to be entirely independent from naltrexone's better-known activity, at higher doses, on opioid receptors used for drug overdose and treatment for drug addiction.

The results of increasing studies indicate that LDN exerts its immunoregulatory activity by binding to opioid receptors in or on immune cells and tumor cells. These new discoveries suggest that LDN is a promising immunomodulatory agent in the therapy for cancer and many immune-related diseases. Naltrexone also inhibits cell proliferation when administered in low doses. LDN can, in addition, reduce tumor growth by interfering with cell signaling as well as by modifying the immune system. Moreover, it acts as an opioid growth factor receptor (OGFr) antagonist and the OGF-OGFr axis is an inhibitory biological pathway present in human cancer cells and tissues and acts as a target for LDN therapy. Several case reports demonstrate notable survival durations and metastatic resolutions in patients with late-stage cancer when administered an average LDN dose of 3 to 5 mg/day. Since prostate cancer is inflammatory, work with your healthcare practitioner to consider starting low-dose naltrexone (LDN) if you have prostate cancer. It is an adjunct therapy and not designed to replace conventional treatment of cancer. As a daily oral therapy; LDN is inexpensive and well-tolerated. It is a compounded medication in this lower dosage form.

Side Effects: Potential short-term side effects of LDN include insomnia, vivid dreams, fatigue, loss of appetite, nausea, hair thinning, mood swing, and mild disorientation. Insomnia is the most common possible side effect which for many people resolves after the first night. Potential long-term side effects are very rare and include possible liver and kidney toxicity, possible tolerance to the beneficial rebound effect, and other unknown consequences. You cannot take LDN if you have acute hepatitis, liver failure, or have recent or current opioid use or if you abuse alcohol.

Metformin. Metformin is a medication that is used to treat insulin resistance and diabetes. Metformin has been shown to have beneficial activity against prostate cancer. Metformin depletes the body of coenzyme Q-10 along with some of the B vitamins. If your doctor elects to start you on Metformin, make sure that you also start coenzyme Q-10 100 mg a day along with B complex twice a day.

Nutrients. Lower vitamin D blood levels may increase the risk of developing prostate cancer. A medical trial showed a benefit of higher intakes and circulating levels of vitamin D. However, you can take too much vitamin D. Vitamin D is a fat-soluble vitamin and consequently it is stored in the body. Therefore, have your healthcare provider measure your vitamin D level and replace according to your lab results.

Obesity. Since obesity is linked to more advanced and aggressive forms of prostate cancer, if an individual is overweight, they may want to see their healthcare provider, nutritionist, or health coach to discover new methods to help with weight loss and for encouragement.

Stress. Data from an animal study showed that repeated stress significantly increases the transcription levels of several genes associated with cellular proliferation, including proto-oncogenes. In addition, studies revealed that both acute (develops quickly) and repeated stress can induce significant changes in metastatic gene expression. Consequently, stress reduction techniques are very important since everyone has stress. The body also requires a multivitamin for cortisol, your stress hormone, to be made in the body. Taking adaptogenic herbs and calming herbs have also been shown to be helpful. See the section on cortisol in Part I of this book.

Prostate cancer is a common cancer. For many patients it is a slow growing tumor. For some it is an aggressive form of cancer. Make sure that you see your healthcare provider to have your prostate examined on a regular basis. The diagnosis of prostate cancer is primarily based on prostate-specific antigen (PSA) testing, and transrectal ultrasound-guided (TRUS) prostate tissue biopsies, although PSA testing for screening remains controversial. As you have seen, newer diagnostic modalities include free and total PSA levels, PCA3 urine testing, Prostate Health Index scoring (PHI), the"4K" test, exosome testing, genomic analysis, MRI imaging, PIRADS scoring, and MRI-TRUS fusion guided biopsies are now being implemented. Furthermore, new therapies are now available to treat this disease process.

TESTICULAR CANCER

Testicular cancer is the most common solid tumor among males 15 to 34 years of age, with an estimated 9,910 new cases and 460 deaths during 2022 in the United States. With effective treatment, the overall five-year survival rate is 97 percent.

■ Signs and Symptoms of Testicular Cancer

The signs and symptoms of testicular cancer include:

- Acute pain in the testis or scrotum

- Dull ache in the scrotum or abdomen

- Firmness of the testis

- Painless, solid testicular mass

- Scrotal heaviness

- Scrotal swelling

Individuals with symptoms of metastatic disease (about 5 percent of patients with testicular cancer) may present with a neck mass, abdominal mass, lumbar back pain, cough, hemoptysis (coughing up blood), dyspnea (shortness of breath), or gastrointestinal symptoms. Approximately 10 percent of men with testicular cancer have gynecomastia (breast enlargement) from tumors that secrete beta subunit of human chorionic gonadotropin (HCG).

Epididymitis

Epididymitis is an important part of the differential diagnosis of a scrotal mass. Epididymitis is an inflammation of the coiled tube (epididymis) at the back of the testicle that stores and carries sperm. If tenderness, swelling, or examination abnormalities persist after antibiotic treatment, further evaluation is necessary to rule out testicular cancer.

■ Risk Factors for Testicular Cancer

The risk factors for testicular cancer are numerous.

- In individuals with undescended testis (cryptorchidism), the relative risk of developing testicular cancer ranges from 2.9 to 6.3; the risk is increased in both testes, although the risk is much higher in the ipsilateral (same side) testis. Among these patients, the risk of cancer increases when orchiopexy is delayed until after puberty or never performed compared with early orchiopexy. Orchiopexy describes the operation to surgically correct an undescended testicle; to move and/or permanently fix a testicle into the scrotum. Even after early orchiopexy, the risk of testicular cancer remains elevated compared with the general population.

- Men with a personal history of testicular cancer have a 12-times greater risk of developing a contralateral (opposite side) testicular cancer than the general population. However, the greatest risk is in the first five years after diagnosis, and the 15-year cumulative risk is 1.9 percent. In addition, patients with a father or brother with testicular cancer have a significantly great risk of developing the disease.

- Moreover, men with infertility have an increased risk of developing testicular cancer, although the underlying mechanism is unclear.

- Associations between testicular cancer and marijuana use, inguinal hernia, diet, maternal smoking, and body size are inconclusive.

- Testicular microlithiasis, and vasectomy are not risk factors for testicular cancer.

- Infections with human papillomavirus (HPV), Epstein-Barr virus (EBV), cytomegalovirus (CMV), parvovirus B-19, and human immunodeficiency virus (HIV) increase an individual's risk.

- In addition, trauma to the testicle is a risk factor. Furthermore, high maternal estrogen levels are also a risk factor.

- However, testicular microlithiasis, and vasectomy are not risk factors for testicular cancer.

▇ Therapies for Testicular Cancer

Conventional Treatments

- **Orchiectomy.** If a solid intratesticular mass is discovered, orchiectomy (testicle removal) is both diagnostic and therapeutic. Radical inguinal orchiectomy is a surgical procedure in which one or both testicles are removed, including removal of the spermatic cord to the internal inguinal ring. It is the primary treatment for any malignant tumor found on surgical exploration of a testicular mass. Testis-sparing surgery is generally not recommended but may be performed for a small tumor in one testis or for small bilateral (both sides) tumors. Orchiectomy may be delayed if life-threatening metastases require more urgent attention.

  Treatment after orchiectomy is based on histology, staging, prognosis, and an individualized discussion with your oncologist and urologist on the benefits and risks of treatment options.

Orchiectomy Radiation and/or Chemotherapy and Their Risks

Infertility and hypogonadism should be addressed. Cancer alone may affect fertility. A systematic review found that up to 50 percent of men with testicular cancer have semen abnormalities prior to orchiectomy. Orchiectomy and the effects of chemotherapy and radiation also carry significant risks of future infertility. Retrograde ejaculation (when the semen travels backwards into the bladder) or anejaculation (inability to ejaculate) may occur, but advances in surgical techniques have reduced these risks.

Adjuvant therapy increases the short- and long-term risks of cardiovascular disease in testicular cancer survivors. A recent population-based study of more than 15,000 testicular cancer survivors found a fivefold increased risk of cardiovascular mortality within the first year after chemotherapy compared with orchiectomy alone. This cardiovascular risk was not significant beyond the first year. A retrospective study of testicular cancer survivors compared with age-matched control patients showed that radiotherapy or chemotherapy imposes greater than a twofold increased long-term risk (after 10 years posttreatment) for atherosclerotic heart disease; combined therapy increased the risk to almost fivefold. Mediastinal irradiation carries more risk than subphrenic irradiation. There are no evidence-based recommendations for heart disease screening in testicular cancer survivors. Patients and their healthcare providers should be aware of potential cardiovascular risk in testicular cancer survivors.

- **Radiation and/or Chemotherapy**. Additional therapies may include radiation and/or chemotherapy. The high survival rate and young age of patients with testicular cancer result in long periods of survivorship with multiple sources of potential morbidity and mortality. Complications arise from both the disease process and treatment and vary according to each individual.

  Secondary malignancy may be a concern. Testicular cancer survivors treated with radiotherapy or chemotherapy are at increased risk of secondary malignant neoplasms. There is a threefold increased risk of leukemia among testicular cancer survivors treated with radiotherapy to the abdomen and pelvis. Cisplatin and etoposide therapies also increase the risk of secondary leukemia. Radiotherapy and chemotherapy increase the risk of solid cancers beginning five years after treatment. Sites of secondary malignancy include stomach, pancreas, pleura, bladder, colon, and esophagus.

Precision Medicine Therapies

Precision Medicine therapies include all the conventional approaches discussed previously along with the following treatments.

Inflammation. One study hypothesized a correlation between low testosterone levels and increased secretion of pro-inflammatory cytokines as the cause and maintenance of chronic diseases. You can lower the inflammatory component in your body with EPA/DHA (fish oil) and curcumin.

Low-Dose Naltrexone (LDN). Your healthcare provider can also prescribe low-dose naltrexone. Moreover, the results of increasing studies indicate that LDN exerts its immunoregulatory activity by binding to opioid receptors in or on immune cells and tumor cells. These new discoveries indicate that LDN is a promising immunomodulatory agent in the therapy for cancer and many immune-related diseases. It has also been reported that LDN is able to reduce tumor growth by interfering with cell signaling as well as by modifying the immune system. This data supports further the idea that LDN possesses anticancer activity. For a further discussion concerning LDN see the previous section on prostate cancer.

Smoking. Stop smoking! Smoking cessation therapies have been shown to be helpful for many people.

Stress. Stress from any cause is known to modify the immune response and can partially suppress certain aspects of immune function. In addition, prolonged psychological stress appears to be correlated with cellular aging, inducing characteristic senescence (process of deterioration with age) features, such as increased oxidative stress, reduced telomere length, chronic exposure to glucocorticoids, decreased thymus, changes in cell trafficking, decreased cell-mediated immune response, steroid resistance, and chronic low-grade inflammation.

Furthermore, both biological and psychological stress experienced during cancer therapy may be responsible for stimulating molecular processes that induce premature aging and deterioration of immune system in testicular cancer survivors, leading to an increased susceptibility to infections, reoccurence of cancer, and autoimmune diseases.

Testosterone Replacement. A recent study is the first to investigate the effect of testosterone replacement in testicular cancer survivors with mild Leydig cell insufficiency. In younger men, HCG or clomiphene citrate may be used to raise testosterone if levels are low instead of testosterone itself. See your oncologist and also a Precision/Anti-Aging specialist to discuss testosterone replacement, HCG, or clomiphene therapies if you have a history of testicular cancer.

CONCLUSION

As you have seen there are both conventional and Precision/Anti-Aging Medicine treatments that are successful for testicular cancer. In addition, review with your doctor the possible risk factors for other diseases that need to be mitigated as you age. The increasing evidence that some cancer treatments may induce cellular senescence and aging of the immune system, may have implications on the development of secondary medical conditions later in life. Testicular cancer survivors have an increased risk to suffer of late adverse events, including hypogonadism (when the testes produce little or no hormones), infertility, metabolic syndromes, neurotoxicity, lower cognitive functions, reduced renal function, heart disease, and secondary cancers. Hypogonadism itself also increases a person's risk of developing metabolic syndrome, including cardiovascular complications and diabetes, which appears to be greater after combination therapy (chemo-radiotherapy). In addition, testicular cancer survivors struggle with higher rates of anxiety and post-traumatic stress disorder (PTSD). Many of these disease processes can be mitigated by a Precision Medicine approach to healthcare.

PART III

Hormone Replacement Therapy

INTRODUCTION

A man's body is designed not to need hormonal therapy. If you are nutritionally sound, not stressed, you exercise, you are not overweight, and you are not toxic, your body will usually make the optimal amount of each hormone at any age. However, in today's world there are very few men who fall into this category.

The good news is we now have the science to optimize the hormones in your body—no matter what age you are. Balancing your hormones is a key component in helping you feel great, including helping you maintain sexual interest and function along with preventing such illnesses as heart disease and memory loss. In today's world you can have your hormone replacement therapy individualized and customized to meet your own personal needs. In the past, the only type of hormonal therapy available was a "one-size-fits-all." Every man, regardless of symptoms and severity of symptoms, received the same hormonal treatment. This is problematic, as you have discovered in this book, since two men with similar problems may have entirely different ailments and more than one cause of their symptoms. In addition, some men have no complaints and do not realize that they would benefit from hormone replacement to help prevent disease. Now, with customizable hormonal therapy, a Precision Medicine/Anti-Aging Medicine approach, you can be prescribed hormones specifically designed for you and you only.

In this part of the book, you will learn more about hormone replacement therapy and reasons you should consider testosterone replacement as well as augmentation of other hormones. Information on how to get started, once you have decided to do so, is also provided. In addition, younger males are not prescribed testosterone if levels are low, because if it is given too early, testosterone replacement can cause infertility. There are other methods of increasing testosterone without being prescribed this medication that will be discussed at length in this section of the text. Furthermore, different types of testing methods that measure hormonal levels are detailed in this segment of the book.

Additionally, Part III will extensively discuss four major reasons why you should consider hormone replacement therapy, and how proper nutrition and exercise can alleviate symptoms and maximize your treatment.

Welcome to this new era of medicine.

WHAT IS HORMONE REPLACEMENT THERAPY (HRT)?

Up until a few decades ago, testosterone replacement therapy was not considered commonplace treatment for males.

Ten Reasons You Should Consider Compounded HRT

1. Bone production (prevention of osteoporosis)

2. Growth and repair

3. Heart health

4. Improvement in sleep hygiene

5. Tailored to your needs

6. Safe method of hormone replacement when prescribed in appropriate doses

7. Prevention of memory loss

8. Reduction of inflammation

9. Immune system support

10. Maintenance of sexual function

■ Compounded Hormones

The best way to ensure you receive optimal hormone replacement therapy is to use compounded hormones. With compounded hormones, your HRT therapy will be made for your individual needs. Your hormones are mixed into different dosages, and special routes of administration are available, depending on what updated research and your personalized biology have revealed. There are even different bases in which topical hormones can be placed, contingent on your physiology, including a special base for testosterone to ensure maximal absorption. Your doctor or other healthcare provider will have a compounding pharmacist make your prescription for you and you only. Your HRT will be made from plant extracts that are an exact replica of your own hormones.

The key to effective hormone replacement, in summary, is individuality.

Fixed doses do not allow for customized, tailor-made treatment. Having your hormonal therapy personalized, at any age, helps you achieve and maintain the optimal hormonal symphony for your body.

THE BIG FOUR REASONS TO START HRT

What does the medical literature really say about hormone replacement and cognition? What does the medical literature reveal regarding HRT and heart disease? Does hormone replacement therapy have an effect on insulin resistance, diabetes, and weight gain? Does hormone replacement influence sexual function and interest? Let's examine each one of these individually.

■ HRT and Cognitive Function

The nineteenth century Scottish poet Alexander Smith had it right when he wrote, "A man's real possession is his memory. In nothing else is he rich, in nothing else is he poor." Your memory is you're most prized possession that God gave you. Maintaining your cognitive function is imperative. There are many things you can do to maintain rapid-fire memory as you age, and one of the main ones is hormone replacement therapy.

Testosterone

For males, testosterone literally equals memory. In men, testosterone levels decline at a rate of approximately 1 percent per year starting at the age of 30. Testosterone levels that are bioavailable (fraction of the drug that enters the circulation and therefore is able to have an active effect) decline at twice the rate of total testosterone levels. Thirty percent to 60 percent of men in their 70s are hypogonadal (diminished functional activity of the testes) and consequently do not make optimal levels of testosterone, DHEA, and/or pregnenolone. The good news for men is that they develop Alzheimer's disease at a rate that is slower than women. The bad news is that with men, dementia has a higher mortality rate. Studies have shown that the development of memory loss in males is related, in part, to the loss of testosterone that occurs with age.

In men, testosterone plays a major role in brain functioning. Subclinical androgen deficiency has been suggested to increase the expression of amyloid-B-related peptides which is related to Alzheimer's disease.

In one trial, age-related decline in free testosterone predicted age-related decline in visual and verbal memory. In fact, low levels of bioavailable testosterone are a positive predictor of memory loss in men as they age. In a medical study conducted in Hong Kong, in men with low bioavailable testosterone levels there was a strong correlation with memory loss/ Alzheimer's disease. Furthermore, individuals with Alzheimer's disease have been shown to have a lower ratio of total testosterone to sex hormone binding globulin (SHBG) when compared with age-matched controls. Moreover, decreased levels of testosterone may occur prior to the diagnosis of Alzheimer's disease. In addition, low testosterone levels have also been associated with mild memory loss. Likewise, lower levels of testosterone may be related to an elevated risk of all-cause dementia including Alzheimer's disease. However, males that have a higher ratio of total testosterone to SHBG have a lower rate of development of Alzheimer's disease. In another medical trial, which was a prospective longitudinal study, it revealed that the risk of Alzheimer's disease was decreased by 26 percent for each 10-unit (nmoL/nmoL) increase in free testosterone at 2, 5, and 10 years before the diagnosis of Alzheimer's disease was made. Studies have also shown a correlation between testosterone levels and cognitive abilities, such as spatial performance and mathematical reasoning. In fact, higher levels of free concentrations of this important hormone have been associated with better performance in specific aspects of memory and cognitive function. In yet another study, optimal processing capacity was found in men between the ages of 35 and 90 even after adjustment for age, education, and cardiovascular morbidity in men that had higher free levels of testosterone. The same was not true of total testosterone levels.

Testosterone replacement aids in memory maintenance by helping to prevent the production of beta amyloid plaques, which are aggregates of misfolded proteins that form in the spaces between nerve cells. They are thought to play a central role in the development of Alzheimer's disease. In addition, a study showed that testosterone therapy in elderly men showed some reversal of cognitive dysfunction and another trial revealed that testosterone therapy has been shown to help with mild cognitive impairment. Furthermore, testosterone therapy in hypogonadal men improved spatial cognition and verbal fluency. In addition, in senior men without dementia testosterone replacement reduced working memory errors. Furthermore, findings of one study indicated an improvement on global cognition with testosterone treatment.

Consequently, it is imperative to see a Prevision Medicine/Anti-Aging specialist or compounding pharmacist to have your hormone levels measured by saliva. If your levels are low, have the healthcare provider start you on testosterone transdermally (applied on the skin), if you are a candidate for testosterone replacement.

Progesterone

Progesterone promotes the formation of myelin sheaths and has many positive effects on your neurons. It also helps regulate brain levels of certain neurotransmitters associated with learning and memory, including dopamine and GABA. In addition, progesterone also exerts a neuroprotective role, which can be effective to counteract the cognitive decline related to aging. Therefore, scientists are now looking at progesterone replacement to aid in the prevention of memory loss. One study found that progesterone therapy reduced the impairment in spatial, reference, and working memory in people who suffered global cerebral ischemia, a condition in which the brain does not receive enough oxygen as a result of a heart attack or stroke. In addition, progesterone was found to prevent the narrowing of the brain's memory center, the hippocampus, which is otherwise damaged by ischemia. If your progesterone level is low, your Precision/Anti-Aging specialist can add progesterone to the same syringe or pump that your testosterone is in. Progesterone can also be compounded separately for you if your testosterone level is normal. Progesterone is also used to lower elevated dihydrotestosterone (DHT) levels and has a lower side effect profile than conventional prescription medications used for this purpose.

DHEA and Cortisol

Low DHEA levels are often caused by stress and the aging process and can lead to cognitive decline. In one study, researchers found that patients with Alzheimer's disease had DHEA levels that were 48 percent lower than those of their normal counterparts. Consequently, if your DHEA level is low, your Precision Medicine/Anti-Aging Medicine specialist will have DHEA compounded for you to take as a capsule in the morning. If you have a history of prostate cancer, this hormone is not for you since it makes estrogen and testosterone in the body. When your health provider prescribes you DHEA, it is important that you also take adaptogenic herbs and possibly calming herbs to normalized cortisol if it is abnormal. Otherwise, if you only take DHEA, the next time it is measured, your level will be lower, even though you are using DHEA, since the body requires more than DHEA to improve cortisol levels.

When produced in normal amounts, cortisol is very useful for the maintenance of memory and brain function. In particular, cortisol helps to regulate the prefrontal cortex, the area of the brain that is responsible for working memory, personality expression, critical analysis, and decision-making. As discussed previously, stress can increase the amount of cortisol your body produces. When you are under chronic stress or long-term stress, your body churns out more and more cortisol in an ongoing attempt to manage the pressure. In addition, cortisol levels commonly elevate with age. This elevation creates a number of negative consequences for your memory. Studies have revealed that excess cortisol can destroy existing nerve cells and even rewire the electrical circuits of the brain. It can also indirectly cause the destruction of brain cells by stimulating the production of free radicals. A trial showed that older men who secreted the largest amounts of epinephrine (which occurs with stress) were more likely to have memory loss. The hippocampus, your brain's memory center, is especially vulnerable to stress; when exposed to excess levels of cortisol, cells in the hippocampus begin to die. Damage to the hippocampus as the result of stress can also lead to memory loss. As a result, high cortisol levels are associated with decreased cognitive function and increased risk of Alzheimer's disease and other forms of dementia and memory loss.

As discussed in the section on cortisol (see page 24), there are many ways to lower cortisol levels and one of them is to replace DHEA if the level is low. Stress reduction techniques are also very important as are nutritional therapies.

Pregnenolone

Pregnenolone is your hormone of memory. In addition to serving as the precursor for other steroid hormones, pregnenolone exerts its own effect as an anti-inflammatory molecule to maintain immune homeostasis (balance) in various inflammatory conditions. Pregnenolone and its metabolic breakdown products have been shown to have other beneficial effects in the brain, including enhancing memory and learning, reversing depressive disorders, and modulating cognitive functions. Interestingly, a study revealed that pregnenolone may protect the brain from cannabis intoxication. Discuss with your healthcare provider about measuring your pregnenolone levels and prescribing compounded pregnenolone if your level is low or suboptimal, provided you are a suitable candidate for hormone replacement therapy. If you have had prostate cancer, this hormone is not one you should consider taking.

Melatonin

Melatonin has many functions in the body as you have seen in Part I of this text. One function that is rarely discussed is its positive affects upon memory. Studies have shown that low melatonin levels are associated with an increased risk of developing neurodegenerative diseases such as Alzheimer's disease. Some symptoms of decreased melatonin are also common to patients with Alzheimer's disease, such as disruption of the circadian rhythm in the body, mood changes, and delirium. One medical trial showed that melatonin levels in the central spinal fluid (CSF) in patients over the age of 80 were ½ the level of younger/healthier people. Patients in this study with Alzheimer's disease had even lower levels, which were 1/5 of those in young healthy people.

In fact, studies have shown a benefit in melatonin replacement in patients with early Alzheimer's disease. For example, melatonin supplementation has been shown to decrease the damage caused by amyloid beta proteins and tau proteins. In addition, melatonin has also been proven to guard against the harmful effects of aluminum, which has been shown to cause oxidative changes in the brain that are like Alzheimer's disease. Likewise, studies have shown that replacing melatonin in the animal model of Alzheimer's disease reduced learning and memory deficits. Also, medical trials revealed that using melatonin in patients with Alzheimer's disease resulted in better sleep patterns, less sundowning (associated with confusion, agitation, and anxiety), and slower progression of cognitive loss. Furthermore, studies have shown that supplementing with melatonin helps to protect against developing Alzheimer's disease. Moreover, in individuals with mild cognitive impairment, trials suggested that patients that supplemented with melatonin (3 to 24 mg) for 15 to 60 months did much better on cognitive tests. Have your healthcare provider measure your melatonin level by saliva testing. Commonly small doses are all that is needed to help maintain your cognition.

As you have seen, replacement of sex hormones and melatonin are important in the prevention of cognitive deterioration in people that are hypogonadal. Consequently, a major reason to consider HRT is to help maintain a strong memory as you age.

■ HRT and Heart Disease

The incidence of cardiovascular mortality is higher in men than in women and gender differences are substantially related to circulating plasma levels of sex-steroid hormones. In adult men, the main gender-related steroid hormone is testosterone. Given the important roles of androgens in normal male physiology, abnormal levels must be considered one of the main causes implicated in several disorders and pathological conditions, including heart disease. In fact, a study showed that hypogonadism is a risk factor for cardiovascular (CV) mortality in males.

Testosterone

Recently, epidemiological studies have identified emerging risk factors, including low testosterone levels, as being associated with cardiovascular disease. In men, plasma testosterone levels fluctuate throughout life and begin to decrease in middle age and continue to decline with age. Decreased plasma testosterone levels in men have been associated with the concept of "andropause." This has rapidly become a worldwide epidemic condition related to an adverse cardiometabolic (a condition beginning with insulin resistance progressing to pre-diabetes, metabolic syndrome, and type 2 diabetes) risk profile. Andropause includes symptoms such as fatigue and a decrease in libido and is attributed to a gradual decrease in testosterone levels. There is substantial clinical evidence indicating that androgen signaling plays a key role for the cardioprotective (heart protective) benefits elicited by physiological testosterone levels in males.

Men with coronary artery disease (CAD) had significantly lower total testosterone, free testosterone, and bioavailable testosterone levels in several major clinical trials. Also, low endogenous testosterone concentrations are related to mortality due to cardiovascular disease and other causes. In addition, a study showed men with CAD that were under the age of 45 had total and free testosterone levels significantly lower than controls. In fact, men with low testosterone levels under the age of 45 were found to have 3.3 times risk of premature heart disease. In addition, a case control study conducted over a 7-year period, consisting of 2,314 men ages 40 to 79 years, found that every 173 ng/dL [6 nmol/L] increase in serum testosterone was associated with a 21 percent lower risk of all-cause mortality. This was after correcting for age, body mass index, systolic blood pressure, cholesterol, cigarette smoking, diabetes, alcohol intake, physical activity, social class, education, and sex hormone-binding globulin (SHBG).

Interestingly, low testosterone levels and the severity of coronary artery disease may be related to abdominal obesity. Likewise, low testosterone levels are associated with an increased risk for the development of type 2 diabetes and metabolic syndrome. In fact, since testosterone has been shown to lower blood sugar levels, the Endocrine Society now recommends measurement of testosterone in all male patients with type 2 diabetes. See the next section in this part of the book for a further discussion on insulin resistance and diabetes related to low testosterone levels.

Decreased total testosterone concentrations are furthermore predictive of developing other diseases related to heart disease, such as hypertension (high blood pressure), suggesting total testosterone as a potential biomarker for increased cardiovascular risk. Moreover, in males with heart failure low serum testosterone is associated with an adverse prognosis.

Notably, a study showed a possible correlation between lower testosterone levels, erectile dysfunction (ED), and conditions associated with higher cardiovascular risk. Consequently, if you have erectile dysfunction, it is important that you see a cardiologist for further evaluation!

A study from the Mayo Clinic in 2018 analyzed the main clinical publications in the last 10 years related to plasma testosterone levels, testosterone administration therapies, and their impact on the cardiovascular (heart) system. Evidence indicates that physiological testosterone levels are beneficial for the male cardiovascular system, while testosterone deficiency is associated with an unfavorable metabolic profile and increased cardiovascular risk. In another trial, serum free testosterone levels were found to be inversely related to carotid intima-media thickness (IMT) and plaque score. Intimal media thickness is a feature of atherosclerosis. Moreover, low testosterone levels have been found to be associated with heart disease in men in yet another trial. An additional study revealed that low serum testosterone levels were associated with an increased risk of mortality independent of numerous risk factors. In fact, serum testosterone levels were inversely related to mortality due to CVD and cancer. Additionally, low endogenous testosterone levels were associated with an increased risk from all causes of mortality including cardiovascular death.

Epidemiologic studies have shown that testosterone replacement therapy may reduce the risk of heart disease significantly. There are many mechanisms by which testosterone replacement is heart protective.

- Testosterone is essential for normal healthy vascular function.

- For all-cause mortality, each increase of six nanomoles of testosterone per liter of serum was associated with about a 14 percent drop in the risk of death.

- Testosterone replacement showed a decrease in HDL-C and lipoprotein, both being risk factors for heart disease.

- In a trial, testosterone replacement has been shown to lower total cholesterol. The mechanism of testosterone replacement decreasing lipids may be due to testosterone's effect on abdominal fat and insulin resistance.

- Another study revealed that short-term administration of testosterone induces a beneficial effect on exercise-induced myocardial ischemia in men with CAD. This effect may be related to a direct coronary-relaxing effect.

- Short-term intracoronary administration of testosterone, at physiological concentrations, induced coronary artery dilatation and increase in coronary blood flow in men with established heart disease.

- Further studies have shown that low-dose supplementation of testosterone in men with chronic stable angina reduced exercise-induced myocardial ischemia. Myocardial ischemia occurs when blood flow to your heart is reduced, preventing the heart muscle from receiving enough oxygen. The reduced blood flow is usually the result of a partial or complete blockage of your heart's arteries (coronary arteries).

- Moreover, testosterone replacement has been shown to increase coronary blood flow in patients with CAD.

- In addition, testosterone replacement acts as a coronary vasodilator by functioning as a calcium antagonistic agent.

- Testosterone replacement therapy in men with hypogonadism moderates metabolic components associated with cardiovascular risk.

- Testosterone also acts as an anti-inflammatory agent by decreasing inflammatory cytokines, such as TNF-alpha and IL-1beta, and raising anti-inflammatory cytokines, such as IL-10.

- Testosterone replacement has also been shown to be beneficial in people with congestive heart failure (CHF). It improves exercise capacity, improves insulin resistance, and improves muscle performances in these individuals.

● Additional research suggests that testosterone shortens the heart-rate–corrected QT interval (antiarrhythmic), improves glycemic control, induces vasodilation, and has anti-obesity effects.

● Testosterone replacement therapy has been shown to improve myocardial ischemia in men with CAD, improve exercise capacity in patients with CHF, and improve serum glucose levels, HgA1C, and insulin resistance in men with diabetes and prediabetes.

According to a 2017 update demography report from the American Heart Association, almost one in three adult men have some type of cardiovascular diseases. In the context of human disease relevance, the International Expert Consensus Panel that convened in 2015 concluded that there is a need for a major research initiative to explore the possible cardioprotective benefits of testosterone therapy. This implies that there is sufficient evidence regarding the safety of testosterone therapy in hypogonadal men and that the direction of future research should be set toward defining suitable therapeutic options for cardiovascular disease that include testosterone replacement therapy.

Dihydrotestosterone (DHT)

Dihydrotestosterone (DHT) is a metabolite of testosterone. It has similar but much stronger effects. DHT is estimated to be three to six times more powerful than testosterone. Both hormones are classified as androgens. DHT is primarily created in the organs where it is used, such as the prostate. The enzyme 5-alpha reductase is primarily responsible for converting testosterone to DHT which has been shown to enhance early atherosclerosis. In addition, as a broad overview, an overproduction of DHT is also known to cause an enlargement of the prostate and male pattern baldness. The higher the dose of testosterone that is prescribed the more it is converted by 5 alpha-reductase into DHT. Therefore, it is important you see a physician that is fellowship trained in hormone replacement therapy to have saliva testing ordered to make sure you are prescribed the perfect dose of testosterone. In other words, if you are prescribed too high a dose of testosterone it does not stay as testosterone, but instead converts into

DHT, estrone, and estradiol, all of which increase your risk of developing heart disease if these levels are elevated.

Estrogen

Estrogen (estrone and/or estradiol) levels may become elevated as men age due to increased aromatase activity (conversion of testosterone to estrogen), alteration in liver function, zinc deficiency, obesity, overuse of alcohol, drug-induced estrogen imbalance, and ingestion of estrogen-containing foods or environmental estrogens.

High estrone and/or elevated estradiol and low testosterone levels have been shown to be associated with promoting the development of an atherogenic lipid milieu. Consequently, elevated levels of estrogen in men have been linked to an increased risk of heart disease. Also, elevated estradiol levels in men have been related to acute myocardial infarctions (heart attacks). In one study, men who had a history of myocardial infarction had high estradiol and low testosterone levels. Moreover, a medical trial showed that elevated circulating estradiol is a predictor of progression of carotid artery intima media thickness in middle-aged men. Normal carotid intima-media thickness for middle-aged, healthy adults is usually between 0.6-0.7 millimeters. Test results showing a thickness of more than 1.0 millimeter may mean you have a high risk of cardiovascular disease. In addition, a trial showed that high estradiol in males was associated with an increased risk of stroke. Likewise, low testosterone and elevated estradiol were shown to be related to lower extremity peripheral artery disease in older men. Yet another trial revealed that elevated levels of estradiol in men were connected to an increased incidence of strokes, peripheral vascular disease, and carotid artery stenosis (blockage of the carotid artery) compared to subjects with lower estradiol levels.

DHEA

As you have seen, DHEA (dehydroepiandrosterone) has many functions in the body, some of which help prevent heart disease. In a trial almost 1,200 men were studied, ages 40 to 70 over a 10-year time frame. Low levels of serum DHEA were predictive of heart disease independent of other risk factors. Furthermore, DHEAS (bioavailable DHEA) concentration was shown to independently and inversely be related to death from any cause and death from coronary vascular disease in men over the age of 50. In addition, low levels of endogenous androgens, DHEA, and testosterone, were shown to increase the risk of atherosclerosis in older males.

Atherosclerosis is a specific type of arteriosclerosis. Arteriosclerosis occurs when the blood vessels that carry oxygen and nutrients from the heart to the rest of the body become thick and stiff—sometimes restricting blood flow to the organs and tissues. Over time, the walls in the arteries can harden, a condition commonly called hardening of the arteries. Atherosclerosis is the buildup of fats, cholesterol, and other substances in and on the artery walls. This buildup is called plaque which can cause arteries to narrow, blocking blood flow. The plaque can also burst, leading to a blood clot. Sometimes the literature uses the terms atherosclerosis and arteriosclerosis interchangeably, but they do have this subtle difference.

Moreover, gonadal, and adrenal deficiencies were shown to be independent risk factors for cardiovascular mortality in men with type II diabetes and stable coronary artery disease. In addition, a study of 62 males with type II diabetes concluded that lower circulating levels of DHEA was associated with decreased activated protein C generation. This plays an important role in regulating anticoagulation, inflammation, and cell death and maintaining the permeability of blood vessel walls. Decreased DHEA levels were also related to higher intima-media thickness (IMT) in people with type II diabetes which increases the risk of heart disease. Likewise, the plasma levels of DHEA were decreased in patients with chronic heart failure in proportion to the severity of the disease according to another study.

Dehydroepiandrosterone (DHEA) and its metabolite, dehydroepiandrosterone sulfate (DHEAS), have been for a long while at the center of interest for cardiologists. Consolidated data show that DHEA has protective actions on the cardiovascular system. These actions are accomplished directly through target tissues, such as endothelial cells, smooth muscle cells, and cardiomyocytes. At this level, they are able to activate a complex group of receptors which modulate important functions, such as vasodilation, anti-inflammation, and antithrombosis (reduces the formation of blood clots). Moreover, DHEA replacement has been shown to have a vasorelaxant drug affect as well as inhibit vascular inflammation, which are known risk factors for heart disease. The sulfotransferase enzyme that converts DHEA into the active DHEAS form is downregulated by inflammation. Therefore, decreasing levels of inflammation may raise DHEAS levels in the body. Moreover, a study showed that replacement of DHEA improved signs of arterial stiffness. Another trial concluded that DHEA given orally may help treat systemic vascular remodeling including restenosis—a section of blocked artery that was opened with angioplasty or a stent that has become narrowed again. The mechanism proposed is inhibition of the Akt axis. Many studies have demonstrated that aging is closely related to the phosphatidylinositol-3-kinase (PI3K)/protein kinase B (Akt) signaling pathway. This is part of the reason that some authors have suggested that DHEA has anti-aging properties. These data support the hypothesis that DHEA could be used as a drug for primary prevention of cardiovascular disease, especially due to aging and potentially also in addition to conventional therapeutic strategies, for the treatment and prevention of cardiovascular disease recurrence.

Consequently, if your DHEA levels are low on salivary testing, and you are a candidate for hormone replacement therapy, discuss with your healthcare provider the idea of prescribing you compounded DHEA.

Cortisol

Stress, anger, and depressed mood can act as acute triggers of major cardiac events. Consequently, it is important to have your healthcare provider measure your cortisol (stress hormone) levels by saliva testing. Abnormal cortisol levels are associated with many risk factors for heart disease including:

- Dyslipidemias (high cholesterol and/or elevated triglyceride levels)

- Endothelial dysfunction

- Hypercoagulability: elevated fibrinogen, high von Willebrand factor, high homocysteine, elevated levels of factor XII, XI, IX, VIII, plasminogen, 2-antiplasmin, and plasminogen activating factor. This means that you have an increased risk of having a blood clot or pulmonary embolism, which is a blockage in one of the pulmonary arteries in your lungs.

- Hypertension (high blood pressure)

- Insulin resistance

- Obesity

- Perivascular coronary artery inflammation

Normalizing your cortisol level is a great way to decrease your risk of heart disease. We all have stress. It is about mitigating what causes us stress that reduces inflammation and lowers the risk of developing heart disease. Stress reduction techniques, a multivitamin, and adaptogenic herbs have all been shown to help normalize your cortisol levels.

Progesterone

Interestingly, a small study using depo-provera (a synthetic progesterone) IM (intramuscular) an average of 17 days lowered apoB, apo A-1, triglycerides, total cholesterol, and LDL (bad cholesterol) in males.

- ApoBs are proteins found in lipoprotein particles that are artery clogging. The apoB-containing lipoprotein particles that are the most damaging to your arteries include not only LDL cholesterol but also remnants of chylomicrons and VLDL (very low-density lipoproteins). All three of these, LDL, VLDL, and chylomicrons, promote atherosclerosis. A growing body of research is finding that apoB may be a better predictor of heart disease risk than long-standing guidelines for "good" HDL and "bad" LDL cholesterol.

- The apolipoprotein A-1 (apo A-1) blood test is used to evaluate survival rate or risk factors for individuals with past heart attacks and peripheral vascular diseases. Apo A-1 recycles cholesterol from the tissues back to the liver for further processing. It keeps the arteries clear of plaque-forming cholesterol.

This trial was preliminary. Natural progesterone would have been a better choice to see if it produced the same results. More studies need to be done to determine if progesterone would be effective to decrease the risk of heart disease in males by altering lipid levels.

Furthermore, progesterone lowers elevated DHT (dihydrotestosterone) levels, and in this manner may decrease your risk of heart disease. Lastly, a small trial using progesterone decreased venous noradrenaline, also called norepinephrine (NE), which lowers the risk of developing cardiovascular disease. Norepinephrine is both a neurotransmitter and hormone that plays an important role in your body's "fight-or-flight" response.

Melatonin

Melatonin levels have been found to be lower in patients with coronary heart disease versus healthy patients. One study showed that in patients with CHD their melatonin levels were only one-fifth that of healthy controls. In addition, patients who have developed adverse effects post MI (myocardial infarction) were shown to have lower nocturnal melatonin levels than individuals without adverse effects, including death, congestive heart failure, and recurrent heart attack. Furthermore, low melatonin levels cause an increase in night-time sympathetic activity which can lead to elevated levels of epinephrine (E) and norepinephrine (NE) which may damage vessel walls. Moreover, atherogenic uptake of LDL is increased by higher levels of E and NE.

Melatonin supplementation, if your levels are low, decreases your risk of heart disease. A study found that melatonin inhibits platelet aggregation. Furthermore, melatonin has been shown to reduce hypoxia (when oxygen is not available in sufficient amounts at the tissue level to maintain adequate homeostasis) and prevent reoxygenation-induced damage in patients with cardiac ischemia and ischemic stroke. Likewise, melatonin functions in cardio protection (heart protection) by acting as a vasodilator (dilates your vessels), free radical scavenger, and inhibits oxidation of LDL-C. The quality of LDL-C that gives it a negative denotation is its contribution to plaque—a thick, hard deposit that can clog arteries and make them less flexible. The MARIA study, a prospective, randomized, double-blind, placebo-controlled trial, used IV melatonin in individuals following an acute myocardial infarction that were undergoing angioplasty. The patients experienced a decrease in c-reactive protein and IL-6 which are inflammatory markers that increases the risk of heart disease. Also, it helped with tissue damage from reperfusion after the heart attack, as well as decreased V-tach and V-fib and attenuated cellular and molecular damage from the ischemia that occurs after an acute event such as a heart attack. In addition, a study showed that when patients are undergoing coronary artery bypass surgery (CABG), their melatonin levels are disrupted during the procedure and for up to 48 hours after the procedure. Consequently, some cardiologists are now using melatonin immediately after the surgery.

In summary, previously considered in the realm of reproductive biology, testosterone is now believed to play a critical role in the cardiovascular system in health and disease. As you have seen, other hormones also have a large influence on both the prevention of heart disease as well as mitigating the risk factors of heart disease.

■ HRT and Insulin Resistance, Diabetes, and Weight Gain

There are many hormones that play a role in the management of insulin. Insulin regulates the metabolism of carbohydrates, fats, and protein by promoting the absorption of glucose from the blood into the liver, fat, and skeletal muscle cells. In fact, insulin acts like a key to let blood sugar into cells for use as energy. Conversely, insulin not working effectively in the body (insulin resistance) is a chief player in the development type 2 diabetes. Insulin dysregulation is also a major risk factor and cause of weight gain.

Testosterone

The prevalence (the proportion of a particular population) of testosterone deficiency increases with comorbidities, such as insulin resistance and type 2 diabetes, obesity, hypertension, and cardiovascular disease, ranges from 30 percent to 50 percent. In addition, the incidence (the probability of occurrence of a given medical condition in a population within a specified period of time) of insulin resistance and diabetes increases as testosterone levels decline. Consequently, studies have shown an inverse relationship between serum testosterone and fasting blood glucose and insulin levels. Likewise, both hyperinsulinemia (high insulin) and low testosterone have been shown to predict the development of type 2 diabetes.

In a study of over 1,000 healthy nondiabetic men, there was an inverse correlation (where the value of one variable is high and the value of the other variable is low) between total testosterone and insulin levels independent of age and obesity. Also, in the San Antonio Heart Study, the researchers found an inverse relation between total and free testosterone with insulin. Moreover, a meta-analysis of 21 clinical reports, which included data from 3,825 men, confirmed that there was a high prevalence of low testosterone levels in men with diabetes and/or metabolic syndrome. Conversely, men with higher testosterone levels had a 42 percent lower risk of developing type 2 diabetes. Furthermore, there are also studies which suggest that low testosterone may, in fact, be a precursor for the development of diabetes or insulin resistance. Moreover, the third National Health and Nutrition Survey (NHANESIII) found that men with the lowest level of free or bioavailable testosterone are more likely to have diabetes. Likewise, several longitudinal studies have shown that low testosterone is an independent risk factor for the development of diabetes and metabolic syndrome. Metabolic syndrome is a cluster of conditions that occur together, increasing your risk of heart disease, stroke, and type 2 diabetes. These conditions include increased blood pressure, high blood sugar, excess body fat around the waist, and abnormal cholesterol and/ or triglyceride levels as previously discussed. Low levels of testosterone are also associated with an increased risk of all-cause mortality and death from cardiovascular disease. Hypogonadism and obesity share a bidirectional (functions in two directions) relationship as a result of the complex interplay between adipocytokines (cytokines that are cell signaling proteins secreted by fat tissue), proinflammatory cytokines, and hypothalamic hormones that control the pituitary–testicular axis.

Biochemical evidence indicates that testosterone is involved in promoting glucose utilization by stimulating glucose uptake, glycolysis (process in which glucose breaks down to produce energy), and mitochondrial oxidative phosphorylation (pathway in which cells use enzymes to oxidize nutrients thereby releasing chemical energy in order to produce adenosine triphosphate (ATP)). ATP is a molecule that carries energy within cells. Testosterone is also involved in lipid homeostasis in major insulin-responsive target tissues, such as liver, adipose tissue, and skeletal muscle.

If your body does not regulate insulin appropriately, one of the many consequences is weight gain.

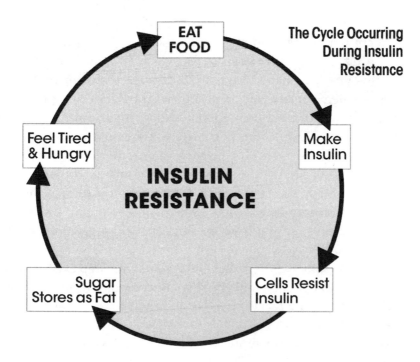

Consequently, low testosterone levels have been shown to be a risk factor for weight gain since testosterone is involved in insulin regulation. Clinicians have explored the concept for years that testosterone replacement therapy helps to regulate blood sugar and therefore helps to control weight. Diabetes specialists have traditionally considered the fall in testosterone level as being a consequence of obesity, but studies now clearly show that low testosterone leads to obesity and metabolic syndrome and is also a consequence of obesity. Moreover, large long-term studies have revealed that baseline levels of testosterone predict the later development of type 2 diabetes. Plus, insulin resistance and hyperglycemia are the key characteristics of type 2 diabetes which are often associated with major weight gain.

Sedentary lifestyle and over-nutrition (excessive food intake) are the main causes of obesity and type 2 diabetes. However, the same causes are major triggers of hypogonadism. Many patients with type 2 diabetes show low testosterone levels while hypogonadal men seem to be prone to become diabetic. Testosterone plays a major role in the regulation of muscle mass, adipose tissue, inflammation, and insulin sensitivity and is therefore indirectly regulating several metabolic pathways. Testosterone replacement therapy is widely used in patients with symptoms of hypogonadism. However, it is not commonly used as preventive intervention or treatment for type 2 diabetes patients even though hypogonadal individuals share many common symptoms (obesity, insulin insensitivity, increased inflammation, decrease in muscle mass and strength) with people with type 2 diabetes. Several studies have shown that testosterone replacement remains a potent intervention improving metabolic functions, such as glycated hemoglobin, blood sugar, total cholesterol, and visceral fat. In fact, clinical trial data are consistent in showing reductions in body fat mass during testosterone replacement therapy. There are also trials showing improvements in insulin resistance and glycemic control with testosterone use. In other words, there is now evidence that low testosterone is closely linked to diabetes and testosterone replacement therapy can improve insulin sensitivity, glycemic control, and weight gain.

Evidence also suggests that a close inverse relationship exists between serum levels of testosterone and the degree of obesity in men. In other words, low testosterone levels have been shown to be a risk factor for weight gain. Obese males commonly have low testosterone levels and testosterone levels tend to be reduced with increased waist circumference and obesity. Specifically, abdominal, or central obesity has been inversely related to total and free testosterone. Vermeulen reported that testosterone levels were negatively correlated with percentage of body fat, abdominal fat, and insulin levels. Another study found a strong inverse relationship between subcutaneous fat mass and free and total testosterone in men with type 2 diabetes.

The symptomatic clinical benefits offered by testosterone replacement to hypogonadal men are well known. In addition, interventional studies have shown the beneficial effects of testosterone on components of the metabolic syndrome, type 2 diabetes mellitus, and other cardiovascular risk factors, including insulin resistance and high levels of cholesterol. For example, the results of observational and randomized controlled studies reveal that hypogonadal men with type 2 diabetes and meta-bolic syndrome attain benefit from physiological (low dose) testosterone replacement therapy. Of note is the consistency of the findings of the four randomized controlled trials of testosterone replacement in hypogo-nadal men with type 2 diabetes and metabolic syndrome. Despite being undertaken by different research groups and using different modalities for the replacement of serum levels of testosterone to within the physi-ological range, all the studies reported an improvement in insulin resis-tance and HgBA1C, along with reductions in obesity and improvements in body composition.

Likewise, a study demonstrated progressive, sustainable, clinically meaningful weight loss in hypogonadal men treated with testosterone for up to 5 years. Many other studies have shown that testosterone is effective, not only for weight loss, but the beneficial effects on waist circumference and glycemic control have been found to be progressive and sustainable. Consequently, testosterone replacement is proposed for the management of obesity in males that have suboptimal testosterone levels. Also, one of the benefits of testosterone replacement to promote weight loss is that it has an anti-inflammatory effect. Obesity is an inflammatory disease.

In other words, there is now evidence that low testosterone is closely linked to diabetes and testosterone replacement therapy can improve insulin sensitivity, glycemic control, and weight gain. Therefore, testos-terone replacement therapy constitutes a valid therapeutic option for men with type 2 diabetes who present with symptoms of low testosterone, which may compromise a significant proportion of the male diabetic pop-ulation. In short, the observational data described above suggest that low levels of testosterone in men commonly coexist with, and that testosterone treatment has beneficial effects on, components of insulin resistance, diabetes, and metabolic syndrome. Such data also suggest that testosterone replacement may also be a valid therapeutic option for hypogonadal men with weight gain in addition to offering a solution for the decreased quality of life experienced by hypogonadal males.

DHEA

A double-blind, placebo-controlled human study provided evidence that DHEA reduced body fat and age-related skin atrophy stimulating procollagen/sebum production. In the animal model, DHEA has been reported to increase not only insulin secretion of the pancreas but also insulin sensitivity of the liver, adipose tissue, and muscle. In addition, other studies have also reported the positive effect of DHEA on diabetes mellitus (a disorder that affects how the body uses blood sugar) in the liver, muscle, adipose tissue, and pancreatic beta-cell and its effect on obesity in animal models. In other human trials, DHEA replacement was suggested to play a role in the prevention and treatment of insulin resistance and abdominal obesity.

It is noteworthy that both testosterone replacement therapy and DHEA replacement have been shown to help prevent and treat insulin resistance, diabetes, and obesity.

■ HRT and Sexual Function/Interest

Impaired sexual desire can result from a wide range of organic, relational, and psychological factors, although it is recognized as one of the most specific symptoms of low testosterone. Sexual interest and function have a great deal to do with testosterone. Current evidence suggests that testosterone replacement therapy (TRT) may improve sexual dysfunction. The most recent large analysis showed an overall improvement in sexual function outcomes in men treated with TRT. In addition, a year-long study revealed that topical testosterone gel resulted in increased testosterone levels and significantly improved sexual function.

Accordingly, low desire has been shown to be improved with testosterone replacement therapy in men with overt hypogonadism. Moreover, in a randomized placebo-controlled study conducted in men with type 2 diabetes, sexual interest and erectile dysfunction improved significantly with testosterone replacement.

GETTING STARTED ON HRT

The fabulous news is that the science is here to help. You can have this individualized kind of medical care. Make sure that you see a fellowship trained specialist in Precision Medicine/Anti-Aging Medicine. These specifications guarantee your healthcare practitioner has completed an extra two to three years of training in natural hormonal therapies. For information on how to find this type of specialist, see the Resources section (page 219). Confirm that your compounding pharmacist has this specialty training as well.

Testosterone replacement therapy has been available since 1939. A commonly asked question is: Does testosterone replacement increase my risk of developing prostate cancer? Studies suggest that testosterone therapy does not increase the risk of developing prostate cancer provided that a physiological dose of testosterone is used. Physiological dosing means the amount of drug given is roughly equivalent to the amount normally produced by the body.

After diagnosing hypogonadism, the currently available treatment options should be considered and discussed with your healthcare practitioner.

Oral formulations containing 17-α-testosterone are no longer used due to potential liver toxicity secondary to hepatic (liver) first pass metabolism.

Buccal formulations have the convenience of oral administration with low potential for hepatotoxicity as they bypass the hepatic first pass metabolism. However, they have a short duration of action requiring 2 to 3 times daily dosing. Mouth-related adverse effects (gum and mouth pain, gum edema, bitter taste, taste perversion) can occur and the clinical response is less consistent.

Intramuscular depot injection (IM) of testosterone cypionate is less expensive and can be administered every 1 to 4 weeks. A major disadvantage is the strongly fluctuating concentrations of plasma testosterone which are at least 50 percent of the time not in the physiological range. This treatment modality also commonly causes supraphysiologic serum testosterone concentrations within 2 to 3 days of injection and a slow decline to subnormal levels within 1 to 2 weeks. This non-circadian type of roller coaster pharmacokinetic response may cause rapid swings in energy, mood, and sexual function. Application regimens of 200 mg every 2 weeks and 300 mg every 3 weeks seem to be effective in moving serum LH (luteinizing hormone) concentrations into the normal range. However, it is not the treatment of choice for most men due to fluctuations in testosterone levels. Some testosterone protocols use lower doses twice a week subcutaneously.

Implantable testosterone pellets are also available but require surgical intervention, may be painful, and are sometimes extruded spontaneously from the implant site. Convenience appears to be the most important factor in the decision to choose subcutaneous pellets therapy, but the cost of therapy is the primary reason for discontinuing it. Furthermore, it is paramount that small doses of testosterone be used if you are selecting pellet therapy. More is not better. As previously discussed, too high a dose of testosterone does not stay as testosterone in the body but converts to DHT, estrone, and estradiol. If levels are elevated of any of these hormones, they can have a major negative impact on your health.

Besides intramuscular testosterone injection, *transdermal TRT* (gel or patch) are the most common formulations used in the U.S. and most of the industrialized world to treat hypogonadism. Several studies have shown that transdermal testosterone replacement is physiologic, efficacious, and has a good safety profile. Transdermal testosterone replacement improves bone mass and lean body mass, decreases fat mass, and improves mood, and sexual function. It also helps lower blood sugar and cholesterol. There are no harmful effects on the prostate if prescribed in appropriate doses. Acne, polycythemia (hematocrit, which is the volume percentage of red blood cells in the blood and/or hemoglobulin concentration are elevated in the peripheral blood), and gynecomastia (an increase in the amount of breast tissue in males) are less common with this form of therapy than with the intramuscular esters. Consequently, transdermally applied testosterone is the preferred method of treatment.

■ Potential Adverse Side Effects of Testosterone Replacement

- Alopecia
- Application site reaction
- Dyslipidemia
- Edema
- Emotional lability
- Gynecomastia
- Hypercalcemia (high calcium)
- Hypertension

- Polycythemia

- Priapism (rare)

- Worsening symptoms of benign prostatic hyperplasia

Most of these potential adverse side effects are related to an over-dosage of testosterone or institution of testosterone therapy when it is not needed.

■ Contraindications to Testosterone Replacement Therapy

- History of prostate cancer in younger males is a contraindication. In older males, the literature suggests evidence for the safe application of testosterone replacement therapy in patients previously treated for prostate cancer with either radical prostatectomy or radiotherapy. Furthermore, there exists evidence that severely hypogonadal levels of testosterone may lead to worse oncological outcomes. The traditional management of maintaining testosterone levels at low levels may no longer be standard of care for these individuals. Therefore, discuss this subject with your oncologist and urologist.

- Presence of palpable prostate nodule or induration

- PSA > 4 ng/mL or 3 ng/mL in men at high risk for prostate cancer without further urological evaluation; also doubling of the PSA within 6 to 12 months

- Untreated severe sleep apnea

- Uncontrolled or poorly controlled heart failure

- Hematocrit > 50 percent (the percentage by volume of red cells in your blood)

- Prolactinoma (benign tumor of the pituitary gland producing prolactin)

- Breast cancer

- Severe liver disease

- Severe kidney disease

Transference is a major concern and has been the topic of FDA warnings. Accidental transference can lead to virilization (development of male characteristics) of contacts, especially in children. To prevent it, areas of application should be covered with clothing as soon as the gel has dried. Hands should be thoroughly washed with soap and water after application. If skin to skin contact is anticipated the area should be washed thoroughly before contact. Swimming and bathing should be avoided for at least 2 hours after application.

Individuals treated with testosterone replacement should be monitored for both treatment response as well adverse effects. They should be clinically evaluated, and their salivary testosterone concentrations should be checked 3 months after initiation of therapy and every 6 months thereafter. If your hematocrit rises above 54 percent, treatment should be discontinued until resolution to a safe level. Your doctor may ask you to donate a unit of blood in order to lower your hematocrit. A hematocrit level should be down to 45 percent and then testosterone therapy can be reinitiated at a reduced dose compared to the prior dose. Your doctor will have you discontinue testosterone and see a urologist if your PSA measurements increase in consecutive 6-month intervals, or an increase of serum PSA >1.4 ng/mL in a year, or if the PSA >4 ng/mL. If the digital rectal examination is abnormal, a biopsy should be performed to rule out prostate cancer.

The clinical response to transdermal testosterone may be variable. Generally, it takes 4 to 12 weeks to restore the serum testosterone concentration to physiological range, depending on the initial concentration of the hormone as well as the type of formulation used. The lipid profile begins to improve in 3 to 4 months, with maximum effect attained in 12 months for total cholesterol and 22 months for triglyceride, high density lipoprotein, and low-density lipoprotein. A decline in fasting blood glucose and HgA1C may be observed after 3 months with further decrease after 12 months. Effects of testosterone on bone mineral density take longer to appear. It may take 6 months to see the initial effect and may take 3 years or longer to reach the maximum benefit. People with metabolic syndrome experience maximum benefit in waist circumference, fasting blood glucose, and blood pressure within 12 months. It is important to monitor your blood glucose concentrations if you are diabetic since you may need less medication for your blood sugar with the initiation of testosterone replacement therapy, otherwise you may become hypoglycemic (develop low blood sugar). Improvement in sexual desire and function as well as mood and energy occur early in the course of treatment, approximately within 3 to 6 weeks.

■ Benefits of Transdermal TRT

Testosterone replacement is best prescribed to be used transdermally (applied to the skin). This form of application is daily and allows for more physiology dosing, meaning that it mimics how the body produces its own testosterone. Intramuscular (IM) testosterone and subcutaneous (SC) are possible modes of administration however they produce highs and lows where initially the level of testosterone is commonly too high for the individual, then it is optimal, and just before the next dose is given is too low. In addition, both IM and SC testosterone therapy have a higher side effect profile than testosterone applied to the skin.

Medical trials have disclosed that transdermal testosterone replacement has been shown to improve chronic stable angina by increasing the angina-free exercise tolerance versus controls that were getting placebos. Another study showed that transdermal testosterone replacement reduced exercise induced myocardial ischemia. Improvements were seen regarding pain perception and role limitation. In yet another trial, testosterone prescribed for application on the skin was 81 percent effective for erectile dysfunction, while the oral form was only 51 percent effective, and the IM form was about 53 percent effective.

The most common and optimal method of administering testosterone replacement therapy on the skin is a compounded gel which allows for customized doses and the use of different types of bases to improve absorption. Apply the gel in an area of less hair such as the inner thighs or the top of the foot.

HORMONAL TESTING METHODS

It is very important to have your hormone levels measured before you begin hormone replacement therapy, no matter what age you are. There are several ways to test for hormones (saliva, serum, and urine), but saliva testing is considered to be the most accurate way to assess bioavailable (the amount of hormone that is absorbed and actually reaches your bloodstream) hormone levels. Hormones are lipophilic, as they have a cholesterol backbone. Because of this, they must be bound to carrier proteins when travelling through serum, which renders them inactive. Therefore, it is paramount that the bioavailable (unbound) amount of the hormone be measured and not the total hormone level.

■ Salivary Testing

Salivary, or saliva, testing is the preferred method of hormone testing for men. It is a non-invasive method of testing and can be done in the privacy of your own home. There are hormone receptors all over the body. For example, there are not only testosterone receptors in the gonadal tissues, but also in the eyes and on your colon. Salivary testing measures your testosterone, DHEA, estrogen (estrone and estradiol), progesterone, and cortisol levels.

You may wonder, how does salivary testing differ from conventional serum testing? The steroid hormones in saliva are representative of the small fraction of hormones circulating in the bloodstream that are bio-available (the portion that is digested, absorbed, and metabolized) to tissues. This bioavailable fraction represents about 1 to 3 percent of the total hormone circulating in the bloodstream. It breaks away from blood binding proteins, enters tissues, binds to unique receptors, and is responsible for triggering specific responses characteristic of the hormone. Blood (serum) levels measure the total level of steroid in the bloodstream, not the small fraction that is released from the steroid-binding proteins in the bloodstream into saliva and tissues, or the bioavailable fraction that is representative of the active level of hormone at the cellular level.

The actual bioavailable fraction of the steroid in serum can vary considerably depending on the level of binding proteins for a specific steroid. This may depend on the level of other hormones and the individual variability in the liver's capacity to manufacture the hormone-binding proteins. Therefore, serum is a much less accurate measurement than that of saliva when assessing functional hormone levels. Moreover, saliva testing accurately measures topically dosed hormones. The discrepancy between free and protein bound hormones becomes especially important when monitoring topical/transdermal or sublingual hormone therapy. Studies show that this method of delivery results in increased tissue hormone levels (thus measurable in saliva), but no parallel increase in serum levels. Therefore, serum testing cannot reliably be used to monitor topical hormone therapy.

■ Blood Spot Testing

Dried blood spot is a form of collection in which you place blood drops on a filter card after a finger prick with a lancet. Once the blood has dried, blood spot cards are extremely stable for shipment and storage. Blood spot is ideal for measuring hormones and other analytes (substance under analysis), such as insulin, blood lipids, Vitamin D, thyroid hormones, and elements like magnesium. It offers distinct advantages over serum because it eliminates the need for a blood draw, saving you time and money. It eliminates needles, fees, and the need to see a phlebotomist. Individuals can collect their samples at home at the time that suits them. Research also shows that blood spot is more accurate than serum for measuring blood hormone levels in patients using topically applied hormones.

■ Urine Testing

Urine testing measures the downstream metabolites, or breakdown products, of the sex hormones, which include many circulating estrogens in the body, as well as other breakdown products. This is advantageous because it helps to make sure the hormones are broken down into metabolites that decrease the risk of disease and not increase the risk of other pathological processes. Hormones in the urine are reflective of the combination of both endocrine production and peripheral production of the hormones and their metabolites

Therefore, urine testing reflects hormone metabolites and is the best medium for assessing the way the body is metabolizing and excreting hormones. Urinary hormones are also a good method to look at the wear and tear (catabolic) versus the rest and recovery (anabolic) balance in the body. If you are in optimal health, your anabolic state is higher than your catabolic state. A high catabolic state ages you, since your body is spending more time breaking down than building up your metabolism. Do not overhydrate if you are taking a urine hormone test because it can affect the accuracy of the testing.

■ Blood Testing (Serum Testing)

Serum measures the "protein-bound," biologically inactive hormone levels in the body. In order for steroid hormones to be detected in serum, they must be bound to circulating proteins. In this bound state, they are unable to fit into receptors in the body, and therefore will not be delivered to tissues. They are considered inactive, or non-bioavailable. If you are using testosterone, which is applied topically, serum testing has been shown not to be accurate, since hormones that are applied transdermally (on the skin) are underestimated in the blood. Consequently, if your healthcare provider uses blood testing to measure topically applied hormones, you can be easily overdosed.

■ Blood Testing That May Be Needed

One kind of blood test that you should ask your healthcare provider to order is sex hormone-binding globulin (SHBG). SHBG is a glycoprotein that binds to testosterone, dihydrotestosterone (DHT), and estradiol. In men, approximately 70 percent of circulating plasma testosterone binds with high affinity to circulating SHBG, 20 to 30 percent to albumin, and the remaining 1 to 2 percent circulates in free form in the bloodstream. Therefore, only a small amount of testosterone is left unbound or free. This unbound part is biologically active and able to enter a cell and activate its receptor. In other words, SHBG controls the amount of testosterone that your body tissues can use. Progesterone and cortisol bind to transcortin also known as corticosteroid-binding globulin (CBG).

SHBG is produced by your liver and then released into your bloodstream, but it can also be expressed in several tissues, including the testes, brain, fat tissue, and myocardium (muscular tissue of the heart). Expression of SHBG is controlled by peroxisome proliferator-activated receptor γ (PPARγ) which regulates energy storage in the body and AMP-activated protein kinase (AMPK) which is a central regulator of energy homeostasis coordinating metabolic pathways and thus balancing nutrient supply with energy demand. AMPK/PPAR interaction is critical to regulate hepatocyte nuclear factor-4 (HNF4), a prerequisite for SHBG upregulation. In cardiomyocytes (muscles cells of the heart), testosterone activates AMPK and PPARs.

Consequently, plasma SHBG levels are influenced by your nutritional state, metabolism, and hormonal factors. In other words, the amount of SHBG that is produced is also regulated by other hormones in your body. Importantly, circulating SHBG levels are strongly correlated with plasma testosterone concentrations and low testosterone levels are strongly associated with metabolic disorders. For example, if your insulin level is too high the amount of SHBG produced is lower so you have more available testosterone for the body to use to help regulate your blood sugar. Hence, individuals with obesity and insulin resistance show reduced circulating SHBG levels. In addition, decreases in SHBG levels are linked to elevated cardiovascular risk factors. Therefore, SHBG levels can be used as an early metabolic and cardiovascular biomarker in men. As you have seen, plasma SHBG levels are strongly correlated with testosterone concentrations, and in men, low testosterone levels are associated with an increase in heart disease. Moreover, a 5-year-long follow-up study indicated that men >65 years of age with elevated SHBG and lower total testosterone were independently associated with an increase of both cardiovascular disease risk and mortality.

Recent evidence indicates that circulating SHBG not only is a passive carrier of male sex hormones but also actively regulates testosterone uptake and androgen signaling. This has an impact on the processes regulated by the sex hormones. SHBG can also release hormones in specific tissues and cells directly, which can influence both production and effects of sex hormones as well as the expression and function of circulating SHBG. Also, sex hormones bound to circulating SHBG can change the affinity of SHBG to its peripheral receptors. Moreover, intracellular expression of SHBG in testicular tubule cells increases uptake of dihydrotestosterone (DHT) and prolongs the expression of androgen-responsive genes.

High SHBG means less free testosterone is available to your tissues that is indicated by the total testosterone level. High SHBG levels are related to lower PSA (prostate-specific antigen) and hematocrit, markers of androgen deficiency. This demonstrates that high SHBG levels can be associated with adult hypogonadism. There are many causes of elevated levels of sex hormone binding globulin in the body as well as numerous medical conditions and medications related to high SHBG.

■ Causes of High SHBG

- Anorexia nervosa
- Aging process
- Cirrhosis
- Diets low in protein in males
- Hepatitis and other liver diseases
- High level of estrogen in males
- HIV
- Hyperthyroidism
- Hypogonadism
- Kwashiorkor disease (protein and energy malnutrition disorder)
- Liver disease
- Medications such as antiepileptic drugs carbamazepine and phenytoin
- Pituitary disorders
- Steroid use
- Testicular disease

■ Medical Conditions and Medications Associated with High SHBG

- Anorexia nervosa
- Hepatitis
- HIV
- Hyperthyroidism
- Hypogonadism
- Kwashiorkor disease (protein and energy malnutrition disorder)

- Liver disease
- Medications such as antiepileptic drugs carbamazepine and phenytoin
- Pituitary disorders
- Testicular disease

If your level of SHBG is too high, eating a high-protein diet may be helpful. Also taking minerals, such as boron, zinc, calcium, and magnesium, may be beneficial. Vitamin D supplementation and taking fish oil are also recommended. Lowering estrogen levels with chrysin will also lower SHBG as well as treating the original disease process.

If your SHBG levels are low, there are potentially more free sex hormones for your body to use. Low levels of sex hormone-binding globulin and is a marker of increased pancreatic beta-cell demand in men. Therefore, reduced levels of sex hormone-binding globulin (SHBG) are considered to be an indirect index of hyperinsulinemia, predicting the later onset of diabetes mellitus type 2. There are many etiologies (causes) of low sex hormone-binding globulin levels as well as many diseases related to decreased levels.

■ Causes of Low SHBG

- Acromegaly
- Anabolic steroid use
- Cushing's disease
- Diabetes type 2
- Excessive testosterone replacement
- Heart disease

- Heart failure
- High levels of growth hormone/IGF-1
- Hyperinsulinemia (high insulin level)/insulin resistance
- Hyperprolactinemia (high prolactin level)

- Hypothyroidism
- Obesity

- Metabolic syndrome
- Weight gain/obesity

◼ Medical Conditions Associated Low SHBG

- Diabetes type 2
- Heart disease
- Heart failure
- Hyperinsulinemia (high insulin level)/insulin resistance

- Hypothyroidism
- Metabolic syndrome
- Weight gain/obesity

If your level of SHBG is too low, how do you raise it? If you are overweight, losing weight is helpful. Also drinking coffee or green or black tea has been shown to raise SHBG levels.

There are other serum studies that are needed to further evaluate your hormone levels. Blood testing is used to quantify complete thyroid hormones. Also, it is important to have a PSA, complete blood count (CBC), dihydrotestosterone (DHT) and pregnenolone level measured by serum.

NUTRITION AND TESTOSTERONE ENHANCEMENT

Proper nutrition, including a healthy eating program and nutrients, plays an important part in maximizing testosterone, preventing disease, and general treatment of andropause. Some of the nutrients you can eat your way into and others you will need to take as a supplement. Exercise is also very beneficial.

DIET

A study found a high consumption of bread and pastries, dairy products, and desserts, eating out, and a low intake of homemade foods and dark green vegetables independently predicted hypogonadism. Therefore, eating a healthier diet with less pastas, breads, and desserts may improve testosterone levels.

■ Magnesium

Several investigations have reported a relationship between magnesium and testosterone concentrations. One study indicated that magnesium supplementation in young healthy men in combination with a four-week endurance training program increased testosterone concentrations at rest and following exhaustive exercise. An additional study conducted on nearly 400 older adult men reported a significant correlation between magnesium status and testosterone concentrations. The mechanism responsible for this relationship has yet to be elucidated. However, it is possible that it may be more indirect than direct.

Magnesium is known to have a role in decreasing oxidative stress and inflammation. Considering that testosterone concentrations can be strongly influenced by oxidative stress, it is possible that magnesium's role in decreasing oxidative stress may provide the stimulus to maintain testosterone concentrations during periods of oxidative stress. A strong positive correlation has been reported between total antioxidative capacity and testosterone concentration.

In addition, magnesium deficiency has also been associated with low-grade systemic inflammation. Low-grade chronic inflammation has been shown to decrease testosterone concentrations by suppressing testosterone secretion from the Leydig cells. This results in both an inhibitory effect on LH secretion and reduced LH sensitivity at the Leydig cell level.

Magnesium also appears to reduce the binding of testosterone to SHBG. Most circulating testosterone is bound to SHBG; however, the bioavailability of testosterone is related to the free testosterone concentrations, which is only a fraction of circulating testosterone. Magnesium binds to SHBG resulting in the blocking of testosterone's ability to bind to SHBG, subsequently enhancing testosterone bioavailability. Magnesium deficiency appears to increase testosterone binding to SHBG, potentially decreasing its bioavailability. Whether magnesium supplementation is effective in augmenting testosterone synthesis as an anabolic agent needs further study.

Causes of Magnesium Deficiency

- Alcoholism
- Caffeine intake
- Diabetes
- Diarrhea
- Excessive sugar intake
- Extreme athletic competition

- Fiber excess

- Foods high in oxalic acid (such as almonds, cocoa, spinach, and tea)

- Gastrointestinal disorders, including biliary and intestinal fistulas, celiac disease, infection, inflammatory bowel disease, malabsorption syndromes, pancreatitis, and partial bowel obstruction

- Medications such as antibiotics (amphotericin B, carbenicillin, tetracyclines, and gentamicin); asthma medications (beta-agonists and epinephrine); chemotherapy drugs (cisplatin, bleomycin, and vinblastine);

cyclosporine; digoxin; diuretics, except those that are potassium sparing; estrogens; laxatives; proton pump inhibitors; and steroids.

- Parasitic infection

- Phosphates in soft drinks

- Potassium or phosphate deficiencies

- Stress

- Surgery

- Total parental nutrition (TPN)

- Trans fatty acids

- Trauma

- Vomiting

Food Sources of Magnesium

The following list is reprinted with permission from *Clinical Nutrition: A Functional Approach* by Jeffrey Bland. MG per 100 grams edible portion (100 grams = 3.5 oz.)

760 Kelp	225 Brazil nut	106 Beet greens
490 Wheat bran	220 Dulse	90 Coconut meat, dry
336 Wheat germ	184 Filberts	88 Soybeans, cooked
270 Almonds	175 Peanuts	88 Spinach
267 Cashews	162 Millet	88 Brown rice
258 Blackstrap molasses	160 Wheat grain	71 Dried figs
	142 Pecan	65 Swiss chard
231 Brewer's yeast	131 English walnut	62 Apricots, dried
229 Buckwheat	115 Tofu	58 Dates

57 Collard leaves	35 Fresh green peas	17 Winter squash
51 Shrimp	34 Potato with skin	16 Cantaloupe
48 Sweet corn	34 Crab	16 Eggplant
45 Avocado	33 Banana	14 Tomato
45 Cheddar cheese	31 Sweet potato	13 Cabbage
41 Parsley	30 Blackberry	13 Grapes
40 Prunes, dried	25 Beets	13 Milk
38 Sunflower seeds	24 Cauliflower	13 Mushroom
37 Common beans, cooked	23 Carrot	12 Onion
	22 Celery	11 Orange
37 Barley	21 Beef	11 Iceberg lettuce
36 Dandelion greens	20 Asparagus	9 Plum
36 Garlic	19 Chicken	8 Apple
35 Raisins	18 Green pepper	

■ Pomegranate and Cacao

In medical trials, pomegranate and cacao (the beans used to make chocolate), improved erectile function and athletic performance. Scientists are of the belief that these benefits are related to higher testosterone levels. Researchers gave healthy males pomegranate for two weeks. Testosterone levels rose by 23 percent to 27 percent, also improving mood and sense of well- being. In animal studies, pomegranate and cacao seed extract were shown to boost testosterone production by the cells of the testes. In another animal study, the combination elevated testosterone levels by over 72 percent in six weeks. In a human trial, men ages 36 to 55 were given 400 mg of a pomegranate and cacao blend daily. After two months, levels of bioavailable free testosterone were 48 percent higher. In addition, markers of stress, well-being, hand grip strength, and low testosterone symptoms all markedly improved. In younger males ages 21 to 35, free testosterone was increased by almost 25 percent. Hand grip strength and upper arm circumference also increased.

■ Vitamin B6

By stimulating the androgen receptors in your body, vitamin B6 signals the testicles to produce more testosterone. Certain medications can cause a deficiency of this important vitamin. Also, cigarette smoking, excessive exercise, food additives (FDC yellow #5), and some pesticides have been associated with a decrease in vitamin B6 in the body. It is always best to take a B complex twice a day, instead of just one B vitamin, unless otherwise instructed by your healthcare provider.

Food Sources of Vitamin B6

The following are food sources of Vitamin B6 from most to least:

- Yeast (brewers)
- Sunflower seeds
- Wheat germ (toasted)
- Tuna (flesh)
- Liver (beef)
- Soybeans (dry)
- Liver (chicken)
- Walnuts
- Salmon (fresh)
- Trout (fresh)
- Liver (calf)
- Mackerel (fresh)
- Liver (pork)
- Soybean flour
- Lentils (dry)
- Lima beans (dry)
- Buckwheat flour

- Black-eyed peas (dry)
- Navy beans (dry)
- Brown rice
- Hazelnuts
- Garbanzos (dry)
- Pinto beans (dry)
- Bananas
- Pork
- Albacore (fresh)
- Halibut (fresh)
- Kidneys (beef)
- Avocados
- Kidneys (veal)
- Whole-wheat flour
- Chestnuts (fresh)
- Egg yolks
- Kale
- Rye flour

- Spinach
- Turnip greens
- Peppers (sweet)
- Heart (beef)
- Potatoes
- Prunes
- Raisins
- Sardines
- Brussels sprouts
- Elderberries
- Perch (fresh)
- Cod (fresh)
- Barley
- Camembert cheese
- Sweet potatoes
- Cauliflower
- Popcorn (popped)
- Red cabbage
- Leeks

◼ Vitamin A

Vitamin A has an important role in testosterone production. A bigger concentration of vitamin A in the testicles increases the excretion of testosterone. Vitamin A also reduces the production of estrogen.

Food Sources of Vitamin A

The following are food sources of vitamin A from most to least:

- Liver (lamb)
- Liver (beef)
- Liver (calf)
- Peppers (red chili)
- Dandelion greens
- Liver (chicken)
- Carrots,
- Apricots (dried)
- Collard greens
- Kale
- Sweet potatoes
- Parsley
- Spinach
- Turnip greens
- Mustard greens
- Swiss chard
- Beet greens
- Chives
- Butternut squash

- Watercress
- Mangos
- Peppers (sweet, red)
- Hubbard squash
- Cantaloupe
- Butter
- Endive
- Apricots
- Broccoli spears
- Whitefish
- Green onions
- Romaine lettuce
- Papayas
- Nectarines
- Prunes
- Pumpkin
- Swordfish
- Cream (whipping)

- Peaches
- Acorn squash,
- Eggs
- Chicken
- Cherries (sour red)
- Butterhead lettuce
- Asparagus
- Tomatoes
- Peppers (green chili)
- Green peas
- Elderberries
- Watermelon
- Rutabagas
- Brussels sprouts
- Okra
- Yellow cornmeal
- Yellow squash

◼ Vitamin D

Vitamin D receptors are present on the Leydig cells within the testes, where the synthesis of testosterone from cholesterol occurs, suggesting an important role of vitamin D on testosterone synthesis. Men with vitamin D deficiency have exhibited significantly lower testosterone concentrations compared to men with normal vitamin D concentrations. Most of the vitamin D you get is from the sun. Consequently, inadequate exposure to the sun can cause a deficiency along with the aging process, some medications, decreased fat absorption as a result of short bowel syndrome or sprue, and sunscreen use. You can get toxic in vitamin D, therefore have your healthcare provider measure your levels.

Food Sources of Vitamin D

The following are food sources of vitamin D from most to least:

- Sardines (canned)
- Butter
- Milk (fortified)
- Salmon
- Sunflower seeds
- Mushrooms
- Tuna
- Liver
- Natural cheese
- Shrimp
- Eggs

◼ Zinc

The physiological role of zinc regarding testosterone biology is related to its requirement in the synthesis and secretion of luteinizing hormone (LH). As previously discussed, LH stimulates testosterone synthesis in the Leydig cells. Zinc is also important in the conversion of testosterone to DHT. DHT has a vital role in the sexual development of males and sexual differentiation of organs. It also promotes body, facial, and pubic hair growth. At elevated levels, DHT increases prostate growth and male pattern baldness. Zinc also has an indirect role in testosterone synthesis. ACE, a zinc-containing enzyme, is reported to increase LH production in pituitary, thus impacting androgen production. Furthermore, zinc deficiency can impair testosterone synthesis and has been demonstrated to correlate with reductions in testosterone concentrations. There are many reasons that you may have low zinc levels.

Causes of Zinc Deficiency

- Aging (zinc absorption decreases with age)
- Anorexia nervosa
- Celiac disease
- Alcoholism

- Chronic renal failure
- Cirrhosis
- Cystic fibrosis
- Hemolytic anemia
- HIV/AIDS
- Increased calcium ingestion
- Infection
- Inflammatory bowel disease
- Iron supplementation
- Medications
  - Benazepril
  - Benzothiazine
  - Bumetanide
  - Captopril
  - Chlorothiazide
  - Chlorthalidone
  - Cholestyramine
  - Cimetidine
  - Clofibrate
  - Corticosteroids
  - Enalapril
  - Ethacrynic acid
  - Ethambutol
  - Famotidine
  - Fenofibrate
  - Fosinopril
  - Furosemide
  - Hydrochlorothiazide
  - Hydroflumethiazide
  - Indapamide
  - Lisinopril
  - Methyclothiazide
  - Metolazone
  - Moexipril
  - Nevirapine
  - Nizatidine
  - Penicillamine
  - Polythiazide
  - Quinapril
  - Quinethazone
  - Ramipril
  - Ranitidine
  - Tetracycline
  - Torsemide
  - Trandolapril
  - Triamterene
  - Trichlormethiazide
  - Valproic acid
  - Zidovudine
- Nephrotic syndrome
- Pancreatic insufficiency
- Pancreatitis
- Rheumatoid arthritis
- Short bowel syndrome
- Smoking
- Surgery

Food Sources of Zinc

The following list is reprinted with permission from Jeffrey Bland's *Clinical Nutrition: A Functional Approach*. Foods that contain the most zinc are listed first, followed by foods that contain progressively less zinc. The number to the left of each food describes how many milligrams of zinc are in 100 grams (3.5 ounces) of that food. Black pepper, paprika, mustard, chili powder, thyme, and cinnamon are not included on the list but are also high in zinc.

148.7 Fresh oysters	3.0 Walnuts	0.4 Black beans
6.8 Ginger root	2.9 Sardines	0.4 Raw milk
5.6 Ground round steak	2.6 Chicken	0.4 Pork chops
	2.5 Buckwheat	0.4 Corn
5.3 Lamb chops	2.4 Hazel nuts	0.3 Grape juice
4.5 Pecans	1.9 Clams	0.3 Olive oil
4.2 Split peas, dry	1.7 Anchovies	0.3 Cauliflower
4.2 Brazil nuts	1.7 Tuna	0.2 Spinach
3.9 Beef liver	1.7 Haddock	0.2 Cabbage
3.5 Nonfat dry milk	1.6 Green peas	0.2 Lentils
3.5 Egg yolk	1.5 Shrimp	0.2 Butter
3.2 Whole wheat	1.2 Turnips	0.2 Lettuce
3.2 Rye	0.9 Parsley	0.1 Cucumber
3.2 Oats	0.9 Potatoes	0.1 Yams
3.2 Peanuts	0.6 Garlic	0.1 Tangerine
3.1 Lima beans	0.5 Whole wheat bread	0.1 String beans
3.1 Soy lecithin		
3.1 Almonds		

Another study demonstrated that using zinc supplementation will not raise your testosterone levels if you are already getting enough of this important mineral.

NATURAL THERAPIES TO INCREASE TESTOSTERONE AND SUPPRESS ESTROGEN	
Supplements	**Considerations**
Antioxidants	Supports testosterone production by decreasing oxidative damage to tissues synthesizing testosterone.
Chrysin	Natural aromatase inhibitor; extracted from various plants, found in high concentrations in honey
Isothiocyanates/ Glucosinolates	Found in cruciferous vegetables as well as mustard and horseradish. Act as antioxidants and inducers of proteins that may suppress prostate cancer.
L-Carnitine	An amino acid that may be more active than testosterone in aging men with sexual dysfunction and depression caused by androgen deficiency. Have your TMAO level measured before supplementing. If it is elevated, do not take L-carnitine.
Muira puama	Derived from Ptychopetalum olacoides shrub in Brazil. Considered an aphrodisiac and effective treatment of impotence by some cultures.
Quercetin	Found in wine and in many fruits, vegetables, leaves, seeds, grains, capers, red onions, and kale. It inhibits synthesis of estrogen by inhibiting aromatase.
Saw palmetto and nettle extracts	Reduces symptoms of BPH. Saw palmetto decreases nocturnal urinary urgency, increases urinary flow rate, decreases residual urine volume in the bladder, and reduces discomfort from urination symptoms. Nettle root may increase free testosterone levels by binding to SHBG.

■ Exercise

Numerous studies have shown the positive effect that exercise has on testosterone levels in men. Testosterone is an important modulator of muscle mass in both men and women and acute increases in testosterone can be induced by resistance exercise. In one study, serum total testosterone levels in individuals with erectile dysfunction, were increased by reducing fat percentage and improving cardiorespiratory fitness via aerobic exercise. Furthermore, in other trials, the combination of exercise and testosterone replacement therapy showed significant improvements in serum testosterone levels and hypogonadism symptoms compared to testosterone alone. In addition, these improvements were maintained in the combination group with continuous exercise, even after cessation of testosterone. However, if you aggressively exercise daily, you can lower your testosterone levels. Interestingly, the Exercise-Hypogonadal Male Condition (EHMC) has been described to occur in athletes who experience low serum testosterone and associated symptoms. This occurs when high volumes of endurance exercise lead to reduced concentrations of testosterone in men. This is commonly a mitochondrial issue. Refueling the mitochondria, with nutritional support, commonly improves testosterone levels without the use of medication if you are aggressively exercising. The following are nutrients for mitochondria enhancement.

Daily Nutrients to Support the Mitochondria

- Alpha lipoic acid: 300 to 400 mg

- Coenzyme Q-10: 300 to 400 mg

- D-ribose: 5 grams three times a day

- L-carnitine: 2,000 mg. Take only if you have a normal TMAO level.

- Magnesium glycinate: 400 to 600 mg

- NADH: 10 mg twice a day

These are doses for individuals with normal renal (kidney) and hepatic (liver) function.

CONCLUSION

Eating a healthy diet along with taking nutrients are both important for testosterone production, as is a good exercise program. In addition, as you have seen in part III of this book, there are many advantages to hormone replacement therapy. Testosterone replacement can, if you have low testosterone, build muscle mass, lose weight, and feel better overall, including improving your sex life. It helps you maintain memory, vision, and mobility as well as assists in the prevention of heart disease and lowers your blood sugar. The testosterone replacement I am referring to is prescription compounded, individualized care, in physiological levels that are equal to what a 25- to 35-year-old man would experience in his life. This is not supraphysiological doses that can cause disease. Hormone replacement therapy is a treatment that should be considered by all men who are candidates for hormone replacement as they age. This decision should be made in conjunction with the advice of your health-care provider, your pharmacist, and a specialist in Precision Medicine/ Anti-Aging Medicine.

Resources

In this book, I've tried to provide all the information you need to create a program that will help you achieve and maintain the maximum immunity. Although you can put together and follow this regimen on your own, it is often helpful to work with a personalized medicine specialist and/ or compounding pharmacist who can customize your program to your special needs. This can be especially important if you are managing a health condition and are already taking various medications. As you have learned in this book, certain diagnostic tests can also be valuable in helping you be healthy and stay healthy, finding the cause of your symptoms, and aiding your healthcare professional in developing a personalized medicine treatment plan, as well as guiding your supplement choices. Finally, whether you design your own regimen or rely on the guidance of a medical specialist or pharmacist, you will benefit most if you use pharmaceutical grade supplements, which meet the highest regulatory requirements. The following lists will guide you to the resources that can help you realize your goal of maximum immunity and good health.

FINDING A COMPOUNDING PHARMACY

Compounding is the practice of creating personalized medications to fill the gaps left by mass-produced medicine. To meet the special needs of an individual, a compounding pharmacy can provide unique dosages, innovative delivery methods, and unusual flavorings, and can also eliminate allergens and unnecessary fillers. Professional Compounding Centers of America can help you find a PCCA Member pharmacy in your area.

**Professional Compounding
Centers of America**
9901 South Wilcrest Drive

Houston, TX 77099
1-800-331-2498
www.pccarx.com

**Alliance for Pharmacy
Compounding**
100 Daingerfield Rd, Ste 100
Alexandria, VA 22314

(281) 933-8400
info@a4pc.org
www.a4pc.org
www.compounding.com

FINDING A FELLOWSHIP-TRAINED ANTI-AGING SPECIALIST

**American Academy of
Anti-Aging Physicians**
1510 West Montana Street
Chicago, IL 60614
1-773-528-4333

www.worldhealth.net

**Finding a Personalized/Precision
Medicine Practitioner**
ForumHealth.com

DIAGNOSTIC LABORATORY CONTACT INFORMATION

Medical testing now makes it possible to measure your amino acids, fatty acids, organic acids, vitamin levels, hormone levels, gastrointestinal function, genome, and much more. This means that your regimen can be personalized to meet your specific needs. The following laboratories can perform tests to evaluate many important aspects of your health. Before ordering any medical test, be sure to consult with your healthcare practitioner.

Access Medical Labs
5151 Corporate Way
Jupiter, FL 33458
Office: 866-720-8386 x120
Facsimile: 866-610-2902
www.accessmedlab.com

Cyrex Laboratories
2602 South 24th Street
Phoenix, AZ 85034
Phone: (877) 772-9739 (US)
(844) 216-4763 (Canada)
Website: www.cyrexlabs.com

Doctor's Data
3755 Illinois Avenue
St. Charles, IL 60174
Phone: (800) 323-2784
Website: www.doctorsdata.com

Genova Diagnostics
63 Zillicoa Street
Asheville, NC 28801
Phone: (800) 522-4762
(828) 253-0621
Website: www.gdx.net

Genomind
2200 Renaissance Blvd., Suite 100
King of Prussia, PA 19406

Great Plains Laboratory
11813 West 77th Street
Lenexa, KS 66214
Phone: (800) 288-3383
(913) 341-8949
Website:
   www.greatplainslaboratory.com

Microbiome Labs Research Center
1332 Waukegan Rd.
Glenview, IL 60025
Phone: 904-940-2208
Website: www.biomeFx.com

Rocky Mountain Analytical
105-32 Royal Vista Drive NW
Calgary, Alberta T3R 0H9
Canada
Phone: (866) 370-5227
(403) 241-4500
Website: www.rmalab.com

SpectraCell Laboratories
10401 Town Park Drive
Houston, TX 77072
Phone: (800) 227-5227
(713) 621-3101
Website: www.spectracell.com

Vibrant America Labs
1021 Howard Avenue
San Carlos California 94070
866-364-0963
Support@Vibrant-America.com

ZRT Laboratory
8605 SW Creekside Place
Beaverton, OR 97008
Phone: (866) 600-1636
(503) 466-2445
Website: www.zrtlab.com

PHARMACEUTICAL GRADE COMPANIES

You can find many good supplement brands at health food stores. Always make sure you buy pharmaceutical grade nutrients. The following pharmaceutical grade companies offer many quality nutritional supplements. Contact them for full product lists as well as for directions on ordering their products.

Biotics Research Corporation
6801 Biotics Research Drive
Rosenberg, TX 77471
Phone: (800) 231-5777
(281) 344-0909
Website: www.bioticsresearch.com

Designs for Health, Inc.
980 South Street
Suffield, CT 06078
Phone: (800) 847-8302
(860) 623-6314
Website:
   www.designsforhealth.com

Douglas Laboratories
112 Technology Drive
Pittsburgh, PA 15275
Phone: (800) 245-4440
Website: www.douglaslabs.com

Life Extension
5990 North Federal Highway
Fort Lauderdale, FL 33308
Phone: (800) 678-8989
Website: www.lifeextension.com

Metagenics
25 Enterprise
Aliso Viejo, CA 92656
Phone: (800) 692-9400
(949) 366-0818
Website: www.metagenics.com

Microbiome Labs
1332 Waukegan Rd.
Glenview, IL 60025

Phone: 904-940-2208
Website: microbiomelabs.com

Ortho Molecular Products
1991 Duncan Place
Woodstock, IL 60098
Phone: (800) 332-2351
Website: www.
    orthomolecularproducts.com

Vital Nutrients
45 Kenneth Dooley Drive
Middletown, CT 06457
Phone: (888) 328-9992 (toll free)
(860) 638-3675
Website: www.vitalnutrients.net

Xymogen
6900 Kingspointe Parkway
Orlando, FL 32819
Phone: (800) 647-6100
Website: www.xymogen.com

References

The information and recommendations presented in this book are based on over a thousand scientific studies, academic papers, and books. If the references for all these sources were printed here, they would add considerable bulk to the book and make it more expensive, as well. For this reason, the publisher and I have decided to present a complete list of references, categorized by section and topic, on the publisher's website. This format has the added advantage of enabling us to make you aware of further important studies and papers as they become available. You can find the references under the listing of my book at www.squareonepublishers.com.

About the Author

Pamela Wartian Smith, M.D., MPH, MS, spent her first twenty years of practice as an emergency room physician with the Detroit Medical Center and then twenty-eight years as an Anti-Aging/Functional Medicine specialist. She is a diplomat of the Board of the American Academy of Anti-Aging Physicians and is an internationally known speaker and author on the subject of Precision Medicine. She also holds a Master's in Public Health Degree along with a master's degree in Metabolic and Nutritional Medicine. Dr. Smith is in private practice and is the senior partner for The Center For Precision Medicine with offices in Michigan and Florida.

She has been featured on CNN, PBS, and many other television networks, has been interviewed in numerous consumer magazines and has hosted two of her own radio shows. Dr. Smith was one of the featured physicians on the PBS series "The Embrace of Aging" as well as the online medical series "Awakening from Alzheimer's" and "Regain Your Brain." Dr. Pamela Smith is the founder of The Fellowship in Anti-Aging, Regenerative, and Functional Medicine and is the past co-director of the Master's Program in Metabolic and Nutritional Medicine at The Morsani College of Medicine, University of South Florida. She is the author of twelve best-selling books. Her book *Max Your Immunity* was published last year. Her book *What You Must Know About Women's Hormones, Second Edition* has just been released.

Index

Within this index, the term "Precision Medicine" refers to treatments which may include botanical, nutritional, dietary, acupuncture, and stress management therapies." Conventional" treatments may include medications, laser therapy, surgery, and lifestyle changes.

A

Acid-creating foods, 156–157

Acute stress, therapies for
  neurotransmitters, factors
    regulated by, 43
  nutrients to increase adrenal
    function, 42–43

Adoptogenic herbs, acute stress
  eleuthero, 38–39
  rhodiola, 39–40
  schisandra, 40–42

Adoptogenic herbs, chronic stress
  ashwagandha, 31–32
  bacopa, 33–34
  cordyceps, 34–35
  holy basil, 35–37

Andropause, signs/symptoms of, 12–13

Ashwagandha
  benefits of, 32
  function of, 32
  side effects/contraindications, 33

B

Bacopa

benefits of, 34
function of, 33
side effects/contraindications, 33

Benign prostatic hyperplasia
  causes, 82
  medications for, 83
  signs/symptoms of, 81
  therapies, conventional, 82–83
  therapy, minimally invasive, 84–90

Benign prostatic hyperplasia, botanicals to treat
  pumpkin seed oil, 89–90
  pygeum africanum, 89
  rye grass pollen, 90
  saw palmetto, 90
  stinging nettle, 90

Benign prostatic hyperplasia, minimally invasive therapies
  precision medicine therapies, 84–90
  transurethral microwave therapy (TUMT), 84
  transurethral needle ablation (TUNA), 84

What You Must Know About Vitamins, Minerals, Herbs and So Much More
SECOND EDITION
Choosing the Nutrients That Are Right for You
Pamela Wartian Smith, MD, MPH, MS

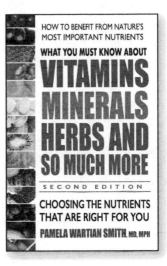

HOW TO BENEFIT FROM NATURE'S MOST IMPORTANT NUTRIENTS

WHAT YOU MUST KNOW ABOUT

VITAMINS MINERALS HERBS AND SO MUCH MORE

SECOND EDITION

CHOOSING THE NUTRIENTS THAT ARE RIGHT FOR YOU

PAMELA WARTIAN SMITH, MD, MPH

Almost 75 percent of your health and life expectancy is based on lifestyle, environment, and nutrition. Yet even if you follow a healthful diet, you are probably not getting all the nutrients you need to prevent disease. Why? There are many reasons, ranging from the mineral-depleted soils in which our foods are grown, to medications that rob the body of various vitamins and minerals. What, then, is the answer?

Now available in a fully revised edition that reflects the latest research and science-based studies, *What You Must Know About Vitamins, Minerals, Herbs and So Much More—Second Edition* explains how you can restore and maintain health through the wise use of nutrients. Part One of this easy-to-use guide presents the individual nutrients necessary for wellness. Part Two offers personalized nutritional programs for people with a wide variety of health concerns. People without prior medical problems can look to Part Three for their supplementation plans.

Whether you are trying to overcome a medical condition or you simply want to preserve good health, this new Second Edition can guide you in making the best dietary and supplement choices for you and your family.

ABOUT THE AUTHOR

Pamela Wartian Smith, MD, MPH, MS, is a diplomate of the American Academy of Anti-Aging Physicians and co-director of the Master's Program in Medical Sciences, with a concentration in Metabolic and Nutritional Medicine, at the Morsani College of Medicine, University of South Florida. An authority on the subjects of wellness and functional medicine, Dr. Smith is also the founder of the Fellowship in Anti-Aging, Regenerative, and Functional Medicine. Dr. Smith is also the best-selling author of seven books, including *What You Must Know About Women's Hormones; What You Must Know About Memory Loss;* and *What You Must Know About Allergy Relief.*

$16.95 US • 464 pages • 6 x 9-inch paperback • Health/Nutrition • ISBN 978-0-7570-0471-1

What You Must Know About Thyroid Disorders & What to Do About Them
Your Guide to Treating Autoimmune Dysfunction, Hypo- and Hyperthyroidism, Mood Swings, Cancer, Memory Loss, Weight Issues, Heart Problems & More
Pamela Wartian Smith, MD, MPH, MS

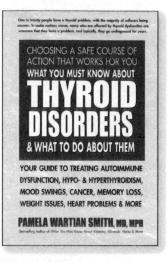

It is estimated that one in twenty people have a thyroid problem, and that most sufferers go undiagnosed for years. But it doesn't have to be that way. Written by best-selling author Dr. Pamela Wartian Smith, *What You Must Know About Thyroid Disorders & What to Do About Them* enables readers to identify common thyroid problems and seek the treatment they need. The book begins by explaining the many functions that the thyroid performs in the body. It then goes on to discuss common thyroid-related disorders and symptoms, including hypothyroidism, hyperthyroidism, excess weight gain, thyroid cancer, and more. Finally, Dr. Smith explains each disorder's cause and common symptoms, diagnostic tests, and both conventional and alternative treatment approaches.

$16.95 US • 224 pages • 6 x 9-inch paperback • ISBN 978-0-7570-0424-7

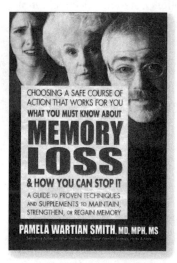

What You Must Know About Memory Loss & How You Can Stop It
A Guide to Proven Techniques and Supplements to Maintain, Strengthen, or Regain Memory
Pamela Wartian Smith, MD, MPH, MS

Contrary to popular belief, not all memory loss is caused by the aging process. In *What You Must Know About Memory Loss & How You Can Stop It*, Dr. Pamela Wartian Smith describes what you can do to reverse the problem and enhance your mental abilities for years to come. You'll learn about the most common causes of memory loss, including nutritional deficiencies, hormonal imbalances, toxic overload, poor blood circulation, and lack of physical and mental exercise. The author explains how each cause is involved in impaired memory and supplies a list of proven remedies.

$15.95 US • 240 pages • 6 x 9-inch paperback • ISBN 978-0-7570-0386-8

Max Your Immunity
How to Maximize Your Immune System When You Need It Most
Pamela Wartian Smith, MD, MPH, MS

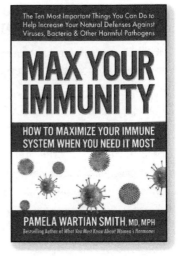

"A guide, written for lay readers. . . an excellent supplementary resource for personal health and wellness . . . highly recommended."

—MIDWEST BOOK REVIEW

The word immunity has unfortunately become an all-too-common term in our vocabulary, and for good reason. When the pandemic hit, many of the major drug companies jumped at the opportunity to create a vaccine that could offer us "immunity" against this specific virus. Yet, few of us understand that almost all these vaccines work based upon their activating our own built-in systems of defense. It is our very own immunity to these viruses that can make the difference between illness and health. To help clarify what each of us can do to protect ourselves and our loved one, Pamela Wartian Smith, MD has written *Max Your Immunity*. Here is a complete guide to understanding and maximizing your natural defenses against various infectious diseases.

Max Your Immunity is divided into three parts. Part One explains how our innate and adaptive immunity systems work. Our innate immunity system is based on our built-in barriers designed to fight or separate us from infectious agents. Our adaptive immunity, also called acquired immunity, is composed of lymphocyte cells that are triggered when a specific pathogen enters the body. These cells learn to identify the invading pathogens and hunt them down. In this section, each component in both systems are clearly identified and explained. Part Two provides ten important things that you can do to increase and strengthen all of these components. And Part Three provides specific nutritional plans to increase your body's immunity to help defend off the most common health disorders.

The fact is, few of us make it a point to keep our immune system in top shape. However when our immune system is weakened, we greatly increase the odds of our getting sick. By simply having a clear understanding of how our internal defenses work and what we can do to increase our immunity; we can play an important role in maintaining good health. *Max Your Immunity* can help show you what you need to know to protect yourself and your family.

$16.95 US • 324 pages • 6 x 9-inch paperback • Health / Nutrition • ISBN 978-0-7570-0512-1

What You Must Know About Women's Hormones   SECOND EDITION

Your Guide to Natural Hormone Treatments for PMS, Menopause, Osteoporosis, PCOS, and More

Pamela Wartian Smith, MD, MPH, MS

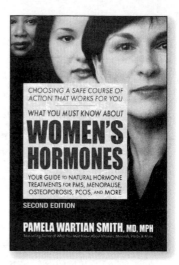

Hormonal imbalances can occur at any age— before, during, or after menopause. The reasons for these imbalances vary widely, and can include heredity, environment, nutrition, and aging. While most hormone-related problems are associated with menopause, the fact is that fluctuating hormonal levels can also cause a variety of other conditions; and for some women, the effects can be truly debilitating. In this new and expanded edition of *What You Must Know About Women's Hormones*, bestselling author Dr. Pamela Wartian Smith has provided a clear and concise guide to the treatments of hormonal irregularities without the health risks associated with standard hormone replacement therapy.

This book is divided into three parts. Part I describes the body's own hormones, looking at their functions and the different side effects that can occur if these hormones are not at optimal levels. Part II focuses on the most common problems that arise from hormonal imbalances, such as PMS, hot flashes, postpartum depression, and endometriosis. You will learn that even disorders that seemingly have nothing to do with hormones, such as heart disease and osteoporosis, can be affected by a hormonal imbalance. Lastly, Part III details hormone replacement therapy, focusing on the difference between natural and synthetic hormone treatments. It explains how you can have your hormonal levels measured, and provides examples of the various hormone replacement therapies available. In addition, there is now a helpful table on the various ways to treat insulin resistance, a key factor in creating hormone imbalance.

Whether you are looking for help with menopausal symptoms or you simply want to enjoy vibrant health and well-being, this new edition of *What You Must Know About Women's Hormones* can make a profound difference in the quality of your life.

$17.95 US • 418 pages • 6 x 9-inch paperback • ISBN 978-0-7570-0518-3

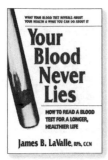

Your Blood Never Lies
How to Read a Blood Test for a Longer, Healthier Life
James B. LaValle, RPh, CCN

A standard blood test indicates how well the kidneys and liver are functioning, the potential for heart disease, and a host of other vital health markers. Unfortunately, most of us cannot decipher these results ourselves or even formulate the right questions to ask—or we couldn't, until now. In simple language, Dr. LaValle explains all of the information found on these forms, making it understandable and accessible so that you can look at the results yourself and know the significance of each marker. He even recommends the most effective treatments for dealing with problematic findings and provides the names of test markers that should be requested for a complete physical picture.

$16.95 US • 368 pages • 6 x 9-inch paperback • ISBN 978-0-7570-0350-9

Magnificent Magnesium
Your Essential Key to a Healthy Heart & More
Dennis Goodman, MD

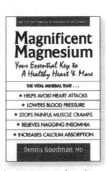

Despite the development of many "breakthrough" drugs, heart disease remains the number-one killer of Americans. In *Magnificent Magnesium*, world-renowned cardiologist Dr. Dennis Goodman shines a spotlight on magnesium, the mineral that can maximize your heart health without side effects. The author first establishes a firm foundation for understanding heart disease. Next, he examines the important role magnesium plays in life processes and explores how a deficiency of this substance can lead to many common health conditions. The author then details magnesium's astounding heart-healthy benefits, along with the additional advantages it provides for other diseases. Finally, he offers clear guidelines on how to select and use this mineral to greatest effect.

$14.95 US • 192 pages • 6 x 9-inch paperback • ISBN 978-0-7570-0391-2

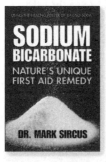

Sodium Bicarbonate
Nature's Unique First Aid Remedy
Dr. Mark Sircus

What if there were a natural health-promoting substance that was inexpensive and available at any grocery store? There is. It's called sodium bicarbonate, also known as baking soda. *Sodium Bicarbonate* begins with an overview of baking soda, chronicling its use as a home remedy. Author Mark Sircus then details how this extraordinary substance can alleviate a number of health disorders and suggests the most effective way to use sodium bicarbonate in the treatment of each condition. Let *Sodium Bicarbonate* help you look at baking soda in a whole new way.

$16.95 US • 208 pages • 6 x 9-inch paperback • ISBN 978-0-7570-0394-3

What You Must Know About Allergy Relief
How to Overcome the Allergies You Have & Find the Hidden Allergies That Make You Sick
Earl Mindell, RPh, and Pamela Wartian Smith, MD, MPH, MS

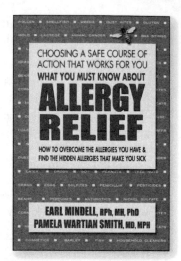

When most people have allergies, they know it. But for many others, allergies and intolerances are hidden culprits that lie at the heart of a number of health conditions. If you are an allergy sufferer or have a recurring health issue that you can't seem to resolve, this is the book for you. Written by a pharmacist and medical doctor, it provides important answers to common questions about allergies—what causes them, how they can affect you, and how you can overcome them. Up-to-date and easy to understand, *What You Must Know About Allergy Relief* offers the tools to identify hidden allergies and the means to relieve their symptoms.

$17.95 US • 288 pages • 6 x 9-inch paperback • ISBN 978-0-7570-0437-7

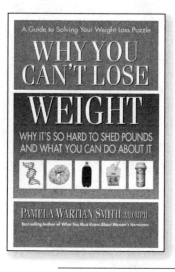

Why You Can't Lose Weight
Why It's So Hard to Shed Pounds and What You Can Do About It
Pamela Wartian Smith, MD, MPH, MS

If you have tried to slim down without success, it may not be your fault. In this revolutionary book, Dr. Pamela Smith discusses the eighteen most common reasons why you can't lose weight, and guides you in overcoming the obstacles that stand between you and a trimmer body. It's time to learn what's really keeping you from reaching your goal. With *Why You Can't Lose Weight,* you'll discover how to shed pounds and enjoy radiant health.

$16.95 US • 256 pages • 6 x 9-inch paperback • ISBN 978-0-7570-0312-7